Handbook of

Sports Medicine

and Science

Running

IOC Medical Commission Sub-Commission on Publications in the Sport Sciences

Howard G. Knuttgen PhD (Co-ordinator)
Boston, Massachusetts, USA

Francesco Conconi MD
Ferrara, Italy

Harm Kuipers MD, PhD
Maastricht, The Netherlands

Per A.F.H. Renström MD, PhD
Stockholm, Sweden

Richard H. Strauss MD
Los Angeles, California, USA

Handbook of
Sports Medicine
and Science
Running

EDITED BY

John A. Hawley
PhD
RMIT University, Bundoora
Victoria, Australia

**Blackwell
Science**

© 2000 by
Blackwell Science Ltd
Editorial Offices:
Osney Mead, Oxford OX2 0EL
25 John Street, London WC1N 2BL
23 Ainslie Place, Edinburgh EH3 6AJ
350 Main Street, Malden
   MA 02148 5018, USA
54 University Street, Carlton
   Victoria 3053, Australia
10, rue Casimir Delavigne
   75006 Paris, France

Other Editorial Offices:
Blackwell Wissenschafts-Verlag GmbH
Kurfürstendamm 57
10707 Berlin, Germany

Blackwell Science KK
MG Kodenmacho Building
7–10 Kodenmacho Nihombashi
Chuo-ku, Tokyo 104, Japan

First published 2000

Set by Graphicraft Limited, Hong Kong
Printed and bound in Great Britain
by MPG Books Ltd, Bodmin, Cornwall

A catalogue record for this title
is available from the British Library

ISBN 0-632-05391-7

Library of Congress
Cataloging-in-publication Data

Running / edited by John A. Hawley.
       p.   cm. — (Handbook of sports
     medicine and science)
   Includes index.
   ISBN 0–632–05391–7
   1. Running—Physiological aspects—
Handbooks, manuals, etc. 2. Running
injuries—Handbooks, manuals, etc.
I. Hawley, John A.   II. Series.

RC1220.R8   R85   1999
612′.044—dc21   99–047560

DISTRIBUTORS

Marston Book Services Ltd
PO Box 269
Abingdon, Oxon OX14 4YN
(Orders: Tel: 01235 465500
         Fax: 01235 465555)

USA
Blackwell Science, Inc.
Commerce Place
350 Main Street
Malden, MA 02148 5018
(Orders: Tel: 800 759 6102
              781 388 8250
         Fax: 781 388 8255)

Canada
Login Brothers Book Company
324 Saulteaux Crescent
Winnipeg, Manitoba R3J 3T2
(Orders: Tel: 204 837-2987)

Australia
Blackwell Science Pty Ltd
54 University Street
Carlton, Victoria 3053
(Orders: Tel: 3 9347 0300
         Fax: 3 9347 5001)

For further information on
Blackwell Science, visit our website:
www.blackwell-science.com

Contents

List of contributors

Louise M. Burke PhD *Department of Sports Nutrition, Australian Institute of Sport, PO Box 176, Belconnen, ACT 2616, Australia*

John A. Hawley PhD *Exercise Metabolism Group, Department of Human Biology and Movement Science, RMIT University, Bundoora, Victoria 3083, Australia*

Mario A. Lafortune PhD *Nike Sports Research Laboratory, 1 Bowerman Drive, Beaverton, Oregon, Oregon 97005, USA*

Henryk K.A. Lakomy PhD *Department of Physical Education, Sports Science and Recreation Management, Loughborough University, Loughborough, Leicestershire LE11 3TU, UK*

Brian McLean PhD *Biomechanics Laboratory, Australian Institute of Sport, Canberra, ACT 2616, Australia*

Ronald J. Maughan PhD *Department of Biomedical Sciences, University Medical School, Foresterhill, Aberdeen AB25 2ZD, UK*

Timothy D. Noakes MB.ChB, MD *Bioenergetics of Exercise Research Unit, Department of Physiology, University of Cape Town, Boundary Road, Newlands 7700, South Africa*

Gordon A. Valiant PhD *Nike Sports Research Laboratory, 1 Bowerman Drive, Beaverton, Oregon, Oregon 97005, USA*

Forewords by the IOC

On behalf of the International Olympic Committee I should like to welcome the new volume in our Handbook of Sports Medicine and Science series, *Running*, published in this very important year, the year of the Games of XXVII Olympiad to be celebrated in Sydney.

Running is one of the purest forms of sport. It is one of the first activities that has appeared early in the sports history of cultures around the world.

On behalf of the International Olympic Committee I should like to thank the distinguished group of internationally renowned authorities who have combined their knowledge and talents to provide definitive reviews of the biomechanics, physiology, nutrition and medical considerations of running for a full range of competitive distances.

My sincere thanks go to Prince Alexandre de Merode and the Publications in Sport Sciences Sub-Commission of the IOC Medical Commission.

Juan Antonio Samaranch
Marqués de Samaranch

On behalf of the International Olympic Committee and its Medical Commission it is a great pleasure for me to present this important publication addressed to physicians, physiotherapists, athletic trainers, coaches and the athletes themselves who will greatly benefit from this outstanding reference.

The primary purpose of the *Handbook on Running* is to provide important information that will contribute to the health and well being of runners of all ages from all parts of the world. Additionally, insights can be obtained that can result in improved performance and full attainment of each athlete's genetic potential.

Prince Alexandre de Merode
Chairman, IOC Medical Commission

Foreword by the IAAF

Running is the most basic sport of all and can be practised by almost everybody. To run faster than others over a certain distance has been the most highly praised ability since competitive sport was born. The popularity of running in our time is reflected in the rapid growth of mass road races over the last several decades. Almost every big city on the globe has its own 'city marathon' with thousands of participants.

Although the ability to run is an inborn quality with nearly everybody, successful running is not a universal gift. The elite runner has aquired his/her skills through a combination of talent for running, systematic coaching and a proper lifestyle. But even an athlete at that level has to maintain an up-to-date understanding of how his or her body functions, how to train and prepare properly and how to watch out for signs of bodily strain and fatigue. Such knowledge is also indispensable for the athlete's entourage, i.e. coach, physiotherapist, physician, etc.

The International Amateur Athletic Federation (IAAF), which is the governing body of running, very much welcomes the *Handbook on Running* to which highly ranked international scientists and experts from various fields of importance for running have contributed. This comprehensive book should offer an excellent opportunity for all concerned to make running safer and better at all levels.

Arne Ljungqvist MD
IAAF Vice President and
Chairman of the IAAF Medical Committee

Preface

I wish to acknowledge the Medical Commission of the International Olympic Committee, in particular Prince Alexandre de Merode for supporting the production of this Handbook. I also wish to thank Dr Howard G. Knuttgen for his unfailing enthusiasm and valuable input throughout this project. I am grateful to Professor Ron Maughan for his support, and to each of the contributing authors for their outstanding efforts. Finally, thanks to Dr Andrew Robinson and Ms Jane Andrew at Blackwell Science for their professionalism in producing the final product.

John A. Hawley
Melbourne, Australia, November 1999

Chapter 1

Physiology and biochemistry of sprinting

Physiology of sprinting

Sprint events are defined as those races up to and including the 400 m, with the 100 m being regarded as one of track and field's 'blue ribband' events: at any Olympic Games or World Championships the winner of the 100 m is accorded the title of the 'world's fastest human'. Although many physiologists have defined sprinting as brief maximal exercise typically lasting less than 1 min, the term 'maximal' should not be confused with that exercise intensity which elicits maximum oxygen uptake ($\dot{V}O_{2max}$). During sprinting, the muscles' metabolic pathways provide energy at a rate several times greater than that which could be met by the oxidative systems alone when they are functioning maximally.

In middle-distance and long-distance running events, prolonged periods of time are spent at 'steady-state' even-paced running speeds (see Chapter 2). In contrast, sprint running is characterized by a constantly changing speed with an initial rapid acceleration followed by a subsequent decline in running velocity as the onset of fatigue develops. Maximum speed cannot be maintained during even the shortest sprint; power output in humans decreases rapidly with increasing duration of effort (Fig. 1.1).

In track sprint events, a runner performs a single bout of exercise with little or no consideration about the rate of recovery from this effort. Accordingly, this chapter will focus on several important factors which influence the ability of a runner to perform a single sprint, and also consider those variables that enable the sprinter to perform consecutive bouts of maximal high-intensity exercise (i.e. during sprint training).

Relatively little research has examined muscle metabolism during high-intensity exercise and, when such research has been undertaken, most investigators

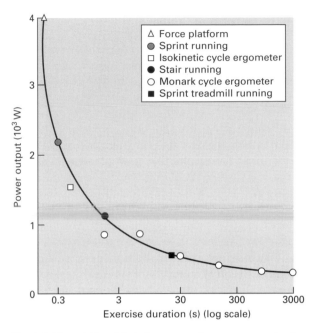

Fig. 1.1 The relationship between maximum power output and exercise duration for various activities.

have utilized sprint cycling as the preferred mode of exercise. This is largely for practical reasons; measurement of power output in the laboratory is relatively easy when athletes exercise on cycle ergometers. This chapter will review the results from the scientific research on sprint running but, because of the scarcity of data in some areas, will also draw from the information derived from sprint cycling studies.

Body composition of sprinters

As far back as 1950, researchers tried to predict how running performance might be influenced by body size. Since then many studies have been undertaken and from the results of these investigations it appears that a runner's height or, more specifically, their limb length, does not greatly affect maximum running speed (the product of stride length and stride frequency). Indeed, it appears that there is a trade-off between limb length and stride frequency: those runners with short limbs cover the ground at the same speed as runners with longer limbs, but with a higher stride frequency. While limb length does not appear to exert a major influence on maximum running speed, the strength of the runner's muscles acting on these limbs certainly does. Although early studies found only poor relationships between muscle strength and maximum sprinting speed, recent investigations utilizing more appropriate and specific tests of strength have reported strong correlations between dynamic muscle strength and sprint performance (Dowson *et al.* 1998).

The influence of strength on sprint performance is the result of the impulse (the product of force and the time of contact) applied by the runner to the ground during the propulsive phase of the stride. There are a number of factors which will influence dynamic muscle strength. The maximum force that a muscle can generate is proportional to its cross-sectional area: the greater the area, then the greater the maximum force that can be produced. Accordingly, if sprint speed is related to muscle strength, then a larger cross-sectional area of active muscle would obviously be advantageous. For superior sprint performance, it is therefore not surprising that sprinters are more muscular and consequently heavier, despite not being significantly taller than other track athletes (Fig. 1.2). Elite sprinters range in height from 1.57 to 1.90 m and from 1.57 to 1.78 m, weighing from 63 to 90 kg and from 51 to 71 kg for males and females, respectively (Koshla 1978; Koshla & McBroome 1984).

Another factor influencing maximal dynamic muscle strength is the fibre composition of those muscles involved in sprinting. The sarcomeres within the muscle fibre are built up of proteins, which exist in different molecular isoforms or structures. These different isoforms create fibres with different functional capabilities, such as different reaction speeds. Muscle fibres can be characterized into two fundamental categories. The most basic subdivision is the characterization of skeletal muscle as either 'fast' or 'slow' twitch, based on the time it takes for the fibres to reach maximum tension. The slow twitch (or type I) fibres are usually associated with a relatively slow maximum speed of shortening ($\dot{V}_{max}$), are adapted for prolonged, low to moderate intensity activity, and are relatively fatigue resistant. On the other hand, the fast twitch (or type II) fibres are able to split adenosine triphosphate (ATP), releasing the energy to 'power' tension development at about twice the rate of the type I fibres. This, in part, accounts for the relatively faster speed of shortening of these fibres, which can be

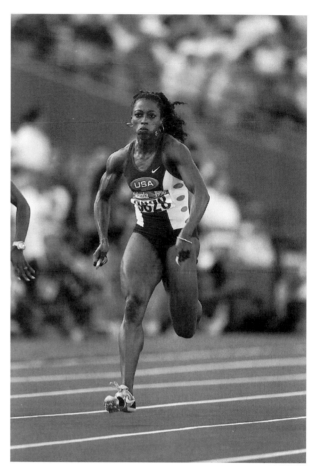

Fig. 1.2 Sprinters are more muscular and consequently heavier than other track athletes despite not being significantly taller. Their leg muscles possess a majority of type II (fast twitch) fibres. Gail Devers (USA) women's 100 m Olympic gold medalist, Atlanta 1996. Photo © Allsport / G.M. Prior.

up to four times quicker than for type I fibres. Fast twitch fibres tend to be larger than slow twitch fibres and also fatigue more rapidly. It is the predominance of one particular fibre type, particularly with regard to cross-sectional area, which determines whether a runner's muscle will exhibit fast or slow contractile properties.

Controversy exists as to whether the two fibre types exhibit different maximum isometric force. However, there is universal agreement that during dynamic movement the force developed per unit area is greatest for fast twitch fibres. During slow movements, both fibre types are able to contribute to force and power production. However, at very high speeds the type I fibres are limited by their $\dot{V}_{max}$ and contribute little to tension development. Consequently, in sprint activities the proportion of the cross-sectional area of the muscle comprised of fast twitch fibres has a large influence on speed. Evidence to support this contention comes from a study by Esbjornsson *et al.* (1993) who examined the relationship between short duration maximum power output and muscle fibre composition in male and female athletes. These workers found that the average power output generated by athletes on a cycle ergometer was related to the proportion of fast twitch fibres within their vastus lateralis muscle. They also reported that the potential of a muscle to generate energy from anaerobic metabolism, based on the activity of two key enzymes of glycolysis (lactate dehydrogenase and phosphofructokinase), was also dependent on the proportion of type II fibres and independent of gender (Esbjornsson *et al.* 1993).

Therefore, it would appear advantageous for sprinters to have a very different fibre type in their muscles compared with endurance runners. Indeed, studies have shown that sprint athletes have up to 80% fast twitch fibre composition of the vastus lateralis muscle. In contrast, endurance athletes may have 80% slow twitch fibres in the same muscle group (see Chapter 2). This muscle fibre composition appears largely to be genetically determined and can only be modified slightly by training. If the relative proportion of fibre types found in the vastus lateralis reflected the muscle composition of all the muscles active during sprint cycling, it has been estimated that the differences in fibre type alone would account for 85% of the difference in maximum power output between individuals (McCartney *et al.* 1983).

Not only is the maximum speed of muscle shortening important for superior sprint performance, but so too is the time taken to generate these forces as the contact time with the ground in sprinting is very brief. In order to maximize the propulsive impulse, force development must be as rapid as possible. The time taken to reach maximum tension in a fast twitch fibre is between 40 and 90 ms. In contrast slow twitch fibres take between 90 and 140 ms to attain their maximal tension. Clearly, fast twitch fibres have a two- to three-fold quicker contraction time than slow twitch fibres

and, consequently, muscles which have a higher proportion of fast twitch fibres will reach peak tension more rapidly, therefore optimizing the conditions for impulse development.

Laboratory measurement of performance during sprint running

In contrast to sprint cycling, sprint running is a weight-bearing activity; therefore there are limitations in using the cycle ergometer as a laboratory-based tool for evaluating sprint-running performance. However, an ergometer for the assessment of power output during sprint running has been developed based on a non-motorized treadmill (Lakomy 1984, 1986). The sprint treadmill allows the runner to sprint at speeds similar to those reached on the track, while also permitting the same instantaneous variations in speed that occur during actual sprinting. Previously, variations in instantaneous work rate during sprint activities were possible to determine only during exercise performed using cycle ergometers, as motor-driven treadmills only have the capacity to produce constant speeds.

Figure 1.3 shows a schematic diagram of the sprint treadmill ergometer. A computer simultaneously monitors both the instantaneous treadmill belt speed and the force being applied by the tether belt to a force transducer. The product of treadmill belt speed and the applied force is defined as the propulsive power. This calculation assumes that: (i) the error resulting in the points of force application (the foot) and measurement (the belt) is small; (ii) the variation from the horizontal by the tether belt, during the stride cycle, does not introduce a large error; (iii) the error caused by the elasticity in the tethering system is small; and (iv) little of any forward lean, which is more pronounced on the sprint treadmill then during free running, is detected as a horizontal force.

Relationship between force, power and speed during sprinting

Often the terms force, power and speed are used interchangeably to describe various aspects of running performance, with the overriding assumption that these terms are describing the same entity. However, during sprinting the runner is constantly accelerating and

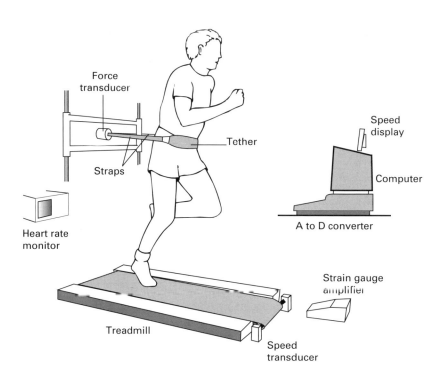

Fig. 1.3 An adapted non-motorized treadmill instrumented for the analysis of force, speed and power output generated during sprint running. After Lakomy (1984, 1986).

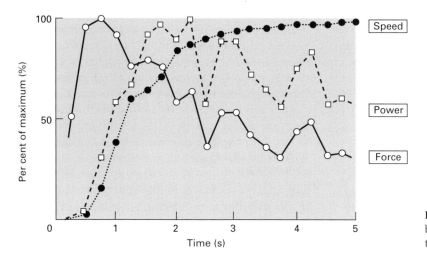

Fig. 1.4 The typical relationship between force, power and speed during the first 5 s of a sprint.

decelerating. In systems undergoing acceleration, there is a temporal link between these parameters such that peak values occur at different times.

Figure 1.4 shows a typical pattern of force, power and speed development during the first few seconds of a sprint from a stationary start. At the start of the sprint the magnitude of the propulsive force is high with both power output and speed still relatively low.

As the runner's speed increases the propulsive force declines, even though power output is increasing. Indeed, at submaximum speed, power output has already peaked. By the time peak running speed is attained, power output and force have declined significantly. During the acceleration phase, peak force is produced before peak power output is reached and, in turn, peak power output occurs before peak speed is attained. This example clearly shows the temporal pattern of sprint running.

Power output generated during sprinting

The greatest power outputs in sprint running are generated during the propulsive phase of the running stride, with values in excess of 3 kW reported (Fukunaga *et al.* 1978). Of this instantaneous power output, approximately 80% propels the runner forward with the remaining 20% of power being required to raise the body off the ground against gravity. Over a complete running stride the average power output can exceed 1000 W during the acceleration phase of a sprint, but this declines rapidly to about 500 W after 30 s.

Energy supply during sprinting

Our knowledge of metabolism during sprint activity has been rapidly advanced by the reintroduction of the needle biopsy technique for sampling muscle, and also the development of reliable and robust laboratory ergometry for the measurement of the power output generated during sprint exercise. The needle biopsy technique allows muscle samples to be taken from an athlete and frozen shortly (4–6 s) after the termination of activity. Thus the samples, when analysed, reflect closely the state of the muscle at the time exercise ceased. This short time frame is very important as the recovery half-time of a number of the metabolic events taking place in sprint exercise is very rapid.

Table 1.1 shows the changes in several muscle metabolites before and at various stages during a maximal 30-s sprint. As can be seen, muscle glycogen content decreased by approximately 32%, phosphocreatine (PCr) by 67% and ATP by 28% after just 30 s. During the same time period, muscle lactate increased 20-fold. These data indicate that anaerobic (oxygen independent) metabolism was the major source of energy to power such a sprint. It should be noted that the fall in PCr is probably slightly underestimated as even the few seconds it takes to obtain the biopsy sample from the athlete's muscle is long enough to allow significant PCr resynthesis to occur.

The data from treadmill and sprint cycle ergometry (Table 1.1) allow us to examine metabolic data for different segments of a sprint. It can be seen that the majority of these changes occur within the first 10 s

Table 1.1 The concentration of various muscle metabolites at rest and after 6, 10 and 20 s of sprinting. This table was constructed by using normalized data from three separate studies using different groups of male and female subjects (Boobis *et al.* 1982; Nevill *et al.* 1989; Bogdanis *et al.* 1994)

Metabolites	Rest	6 s	10 s	20 s	30 s
Glycogen	404	–	357	330	281
PCr	81	53	36	21	14
ATP	25.6	23.2	20.2	19.8	19.6
Pi	2.9	–	14.8	17.4	16.2
Lactate	5	28	51	81	108

ATP, adenosine triphosphate; PCr, phosphocreatine; Pi, phosphate.
All values are expressed in mmol·kg^{-1} dry muscle.

at a time when power output was greatest. Phosphocreatine stores were reduced by approximately 55% during these first 10 s, with only a further 18% reduction during the subsequent 10 s. Thus, approximately 75–85% of the decline in PCr during a 30-s sprint occurs during the first 10 s with the remaining reduction occurring during the second 10-s period (Fig. 1.5). This observation suggests that there is little or no energy available from PCr during the final 10 s of an all-out 30-s sprint. The reduction in ATP stores shows a similar pattern: the majority of the decline in ATP occurs during the first 10 s of a sprint with little further change after 20 s of sprinting. Similarly, lactate accumulates throughout the 20-s sprint with the greatest increase observed during the first 10 s.

It is possible to estimate the rate of anaerobic ATP utilization during sprinting using a formula suggested by Katz *et al.* (1986). The rate of ATP utilization averaged over the first 6 s is approximately 15 mmol·kg^{-1}·s^{-1} dry muscle (dm), of which approximately 50% is supplied by the degradation of PCr. If, however, the average rate of ATP utilization is estimated over the entire 30 s, then this figure falls to about 8 mmol·kg^{-1}·s^{-1} dm, with PCr supplying less than 30% of the total ATP utilized.

The discussion so far has focused on metabolites, or their disappearance from muscle within mixed fibre types. It is important to note that the contribution made to ATP resynthesis during a sprint is different for the two main categories of muscle fibre. The initial

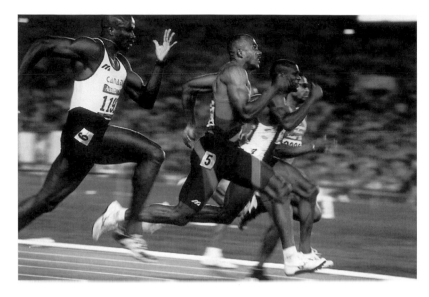

Fig. 1.5 The phosphocreatine stores of the exercising muscles are rapidly depleted during sprinting and are almost completely empty after about 10 s. Donovan Bailey of Canada (left) men's 100 m Olympic gold medalist, Atlanta 1996, and Frank Fredericks (Namibia) the silver medal winner. Photo © Allsport / B. Stickland

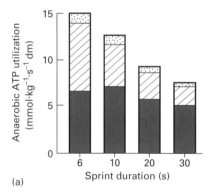

(a)

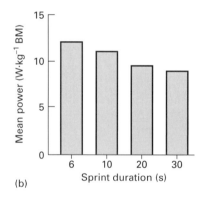

(b)

Fig. 1.6 (a) The utilization of ATP derived from anaerobic metabolism and (b) average power output during sprint cycling for different durations (data from studies cited in Table 1.1). ▦, ATP; ▨, PCr; ■, glycolysis.

stores of PCr and glycogen prior to a sprint in type II fibres has been found to be greater than for type I fibres. Following a 30-s sprint the type II fibres also show the greatest changes in these substrates (94% and 27%, respectively) indicating that these fibres contribute proportionately more anaerobic energy during a sprint than do the type I fibres.

Figure 1.6 compares the average rate of anaerobic ATP production (Fig. 1.6a) and the mean power output (Fig. 1.6b) during sprints of different duration. The rate of ATP production for a 20-s sprint is approximately 50% lower than that for a 10-s sprint, but the difference in power output is only 28% less. Thus, there appears to be a mismatch between the energy

supplied to the muscle and its power output. This discrepancy can be explained by either an increase in the efficiency of power production or a greater contribution to energy provision by aerobic sources during the longer duration sprint. The improvement in efficiency can be observed by examining the power–velocity relationship of muscle (Fig. 1.7).

There is a region in the power–velocity curve at approximately 0.3 $\dot{V}_{max}$ (where $\dot{V}_{max}$ is the maximum possible rate of shortening of an unloaded muscle) in which power output is optimal: at speeds greater or less than this optimal value power output rapidly declines. During a 10-s sprint the muscles are shortening at rates above the optimal speed and so power

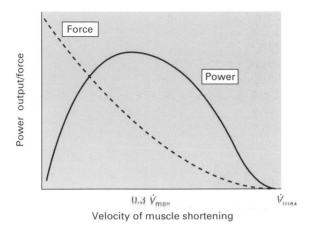

Fig. 1.7 The force–velocity and power–velocity relationship of muscle (concentric actions only).

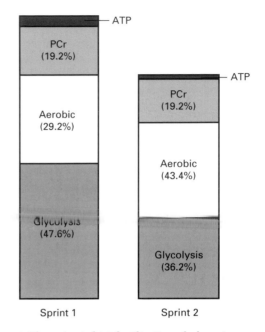

Fig. 1.8 The estimated total utilization of adenosine triphosphate (ATP) from aerobic and anaerobic metabolism during two 30-s sprints separated by 4 min of rest. The height of the column represents the relative average power output of each sprint. Data from Bogdanis *et al.* (1994).

output is attenuated. In contrast, because of the slowing down by the runner the average speed maintained during a 20-s sprint is lower, resulting in the muscles performing nearer to the optimum speed and resulting in a more efficient production of power output. This improved efficiency may account for the apparent mismatch between energy supply to the contracting muscle and the muscle's power output.

It has previously been shown that at least 25% of the total energy required for ATP resynthesis during a single 30-s sprint is provided from aerobic metabolism (Bogdanis *et al.* 1994). In light of this observation, it is clear that aerobic metabolism plays a significant part in energy provision for even the shortest sprint; this contribution increases substantially as the distance of the sprint increases. However, there is a significant time lag between the start of exercise and the aerobic energy system operating at its maximum rate. Accordingly, as sprint duration increases the aerobic power system is able to work closer to optimum while the energy supply from the anaerobic systems, in particular PCr degradation, is severely compromised. This change in the proportional supply from aerobic and anaerobic energy sources can be seen by examining two 30-s sprints separated by a short period of recovery (4 min).

Figure 1.8 displays the estimated ATP resynthesis derived from the anaerobic and aerobic power systems for two sprints. The height of the column reflects the average power output generated during each sprint; it

can be seen that the average power output during the second sprint was *c.* 20% less than the first sprint. As such, the proportion of energy from aerobic metabolism rose from 29% in the first sprint to 43% in the second sprint. This increase in aerobic metabolism was matched by a concomitant decrease in the power contributed by anaerobic metabolism. Sprints therefore should not be viewed as exclusively anaerobic activities. In addition, when examining the data from the first 6 s of a sprint (Table 1.1) substantial lactic acid has been produced in the working muscle. Some of the early literature suggested that exercise lasting up to approximately 6 s was fuelled exclusively by the 'alactic' systems (i.e. those anaerobic pathways which do not produce lactic acid). This is clearly not the case. Indeed not only is glycolysis playing a significant part in energy provision during a sprint, but aerobic metabolism also makes a major contribution to power generation. Simply stated, all the power systems provide energy for ATP resynthesis; it is simply their *relative* contribution that changes with the duration of exercise.

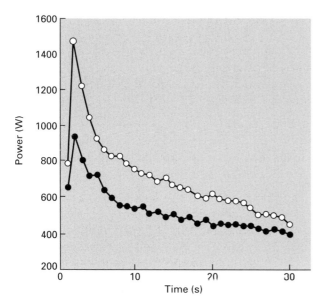

Fig. 1.9 The power outputs of a sprinter (○) and an endurance athlete (●) during a 30-s cycle sprint.

Role of lactic acid and phosphocreatine in energy supply and utilization during sprinting

Although a significant proportion of the energy required for sprinting is provided by aerobic sources, most still comes from anaerobic metabolism. The two main anaerobic sources are the breakdown of PCr and anaerobic glycolysis. In a 30-s sprint, for example, the breakdown of PCr supplies c. 25–30% of the energy for anaerobic ATP resynthesis while anaerobic glycolysis provides the remaining 65–70% of energy. In the final analysis, a runner's maximal sprinting speed is essentially the product of the rate at which anaerobic energy can be produced. Figure 1.9 shows the maximal power output for a 30-s sprint for specialist sprinters and endurance runners.

As can be seen, there is a marked difference in the two profiles; sprinters produce greater power throughout the entire sprint, but also show the greatest fatigue (the difference between peak power and end power output). The capacity to produce energy from anaerobic metabolism would appear to be more rapid in the sprinter than the endurance athlete, but why does this lead to greater fatigue?

Glycolysis is the breakdown of muscle glycogen to form pyruvate and ultimately lactic acid. The lactic acid immediately dissociates to lactate and hydrogen ions (H+). Most of the H+ produced are 'buffered'; however, some remain free. It is these free H+ rather than the lactic acid *per se* which can influence muscular activity. The H+ can reduce the supply of energy from glycolysis by inhibiting the activity of a key enzyme in the metabolic pathway, namely phosphofructokinase. By inhibiting the activity of phosphofructokinase the rate at which chemical reactions in the muscle take place is substantially reduced, thereby decreasing the overall rate of energy supply for ATP resynthesis. The H+ can also interfere with the mechanisms of tension development within the actin filaments. The practical consequence of these events is that the binding sites for the myosin heads on the actin filaments do not become exposed in the normal way, thereby preventing effective cross-bridge formation. The resulting inactive cross-bridges prevent optimal muscle tension development attenuating power output and decreasing sprint speed. The greater rate of glycolysis in the sprinter causes both a more rapid production of H+ and a greater concentration of these ions, which will result in enhanced fatigue by the mechanisms described.

Phosphocreatine stores are rapidly activated during sprint activity, becoming almost completely depleted after the first 10 s of maximal running. However, PCr is quickly resynthesized during recovery: after c. 60 s of rest muscle PCr levels are restored by approximately 50% and by about 90% after 200 s. Therefore, PCr is available to power a subsequent sprint after only a relatively short rest period. In contrast, the muscle pH (an indication of the concentration of free H+) shows little recovery during 5–6 min of rest, remaining at a value of c. 6.8. The prolonged presence of these H+ would continue to inhibit performance in a subsequent sprint. If the restoration of muscle PCr stores permits the continuation of high-intensity exercise while the continued presence of H+ inhibits it, which has the dominant role, and how do these factors affect a runner performing repeated sprint bouts?

By examining the ability to perform a second sprint following different rest periods, the relative contributions of the two anaerobic pathways to the recovery of power output can be estimated.

Figure 1.10 shows the time course of PCr resynthesis, muscle pH changes and the restoration of

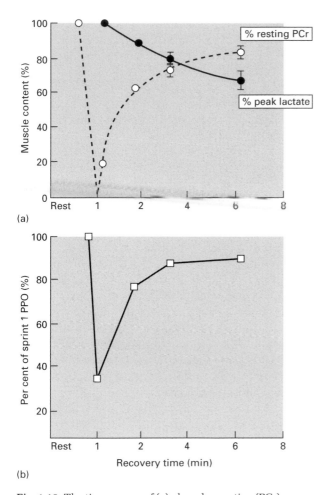

Fig. 1.10 The time course of (a) phosphocreatine (PCr) resynthesis and muscle lactate disappearance and (b) peak power output (PPO) recovery after a 30-s cycle sprint. Data from Bogdanis *et al.* (1996).

peak power output during recovery from two 30-s sprints separated by either 1.5, 3 or 6 min of recovery (Bogdanis *et al.* 1996).

It is clear that the magnitude of peak power output in the second sprint parallels the resynthesis of PCr. Muscle lactate increased to about 120 mmol·kg⁻¹ dm immediately after the first sprint, falling to approximately 70% of this value after 6 min of recovery. The concomitant muscle acidosis, as estimated from muscle pH, remained at the immediate postsprint levels for the first 3 min of recovery and then only deceased very slightly after an additional 3 min. There was still a high concentration of H+ after 6 min of rest. Yet, despite the prevailing ionic concentration, sprint

performance was almost fully restored. This demonstrates that recovery following a 30-s sprint occurs in parallel with PCr resynthesis in spite of the low muscle pH. Accordingly, it would appear to be the resynthesis of PCr that is the dominant factor influencing the performance of repeated bouts of sprint exercise.

Influence of recovery duration on the performance of multiple sprint activities

The previous discussion clearly shows that the length of recovery between maximal short-term exercise strongly influences the ability of a runner to perform a subsequent workout. Training for sprinting often requires repeated sprints (i.e. many bouts of maximum intensity activity interspersed by intervals of recovery). Although these bouts of maximal intensity activity usually last only a few seconds, the recovery periods range from 60 s to several minutes. An important practical question for sprint coaches is how are these very short repeated sprints affected by these limited periods of recovery?

One study examined 10 successive 6-s sprints, utilizing the previously described sprint treadmill, with either 30 s or 60 s of recovery (Holmyard *et al.* 1988). The recovery between workouts had a profound influence on the performance of subsequent sprints. With 60 s rest between sprints, performance was well maintained throughout the entire set, with only a 4% decrease in mean power output between the final (tenth) sprint compared to the first. In contrast, with only half the time to recover (30 s) the decrease in mean power output between the first and tenth sprint was 21% (Holymard *et al.* 1988). When one considers that a 2% decrease in speed, or power, can probably mean the difference between first and fourth place in a 100-m sprint, a 21% fall in sustainable power output is enormous.

In order to explain the large drop-off in performance when recovery between sprints was halved (from 60 s to 30 s) the same protocol was replicated, but using sprint cycling as the mode of exercise (Gaitanos *et al.* 1993). However, this time athletes were given only 30 s recovery between sprints. Muscle biopsies were taken before and after the first sprint and before and after the tenth sprint in order to estimate energy metabolism during exercise. Power output during the first sprint was provided by an almost equal contribution from PCr degradation and anaerobic glycolysis. This single sprint caused a 57% reduction in the PCr store and a 750% increase in muscle lactate. However, by the tenth sprint the average power output had decreased so that it was only 73% of that generated during the first sprint. Interestingly, there was no change in muscle lactate concentration from the first to the last sprint, suggesting that there was very little contribution to energy provision from anaerobic glycolysis. Instead, it would appear that during the last sprint the energy required to produce the power output was derived almost completely from PCr degradation and an increased aerobic metabolism (Gaitanos *et al.* 1993). Clearly, repeated sprints are significantly impaired when recovery is shortened. However, certain training and nutritional interventions can facilitate recovery during such exercise.

Factors influencing the rate of recovery from sprint activity

Aerobic fitness

Resynthesis of PCr and the removal of metabolic waste products following a sprint demand the aerobic pathways and the utilization of oxygen. Compared to sprint runners, endurance-trained individuals have an increased capillary network, a high muscle oxidative capacity and a greater proportion of slow twitch fibres (see Chapter 2). These physiological adaptations result in a faster rate of PCr resynthesis. As the recovery of power output has been shown to parallel the resynthesis of PCr, it is logical to assume that a sprinter's aerobic fitness may influence their ability to perform repeated sprints when the rest interval is short.

The relationship between $\dot{V}_{O_{2max}}$, endurance fitness and the recovery of power output during sprint cycling has been investigated and, not surprisingly, there is a strong relationship between the resynthesis of PCr following a sprint and an athlete's aerobic fitness (Fig. 1.11). Clearly, endurance training can have a significant impact on the ability to perform repeated sprints. Interestingly, an athlete's $\dot{V}_{O_{2max}}$ *per se* does not influence the rate of PCr resynthesis during recovery. Rather, it affects multiple sprint performance by another route; the power output during subsequent

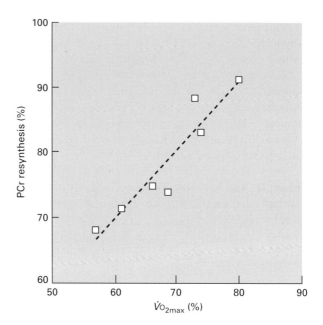

Fig. 1.11 The relationship between the percentage of maximum oxygen uptake corresponding to a blood lactate concentration of 4 mmol·l⁻¹ and the percentage of phosphocreatine (PCr) resynthesis after 4 min of rest following a 30-s sprint. $r = 0.94$; $n = 7$.

sprints are enhanced by an increased contribution of aerobic metabolism. This observation reveals that sprinters with good aerobic fitness compensate for the decrease in energy supply from anaerobic metabolism by oxidative pathways.

Creatine supplementation

A number of studies indicate that dietary creatine supplementation enhances sprint and high-intensity exercise performance in *some* individuals (see Chapter 5). For example, Balsom *et al.* (1993) examined six 5-s bouts of high-intensity cycling and found that creatine supplementation resulted in a better maintenance of power output during the performance of the latter bouts of exercise compared to when the same subjects ingested a placebo. It was suggested that the mechanisms responsible for the improvement in sprint performance were a combination of the higher initial muscle creatine phosphate content, providing more energy for ATP resynthesis during exercise, and an increased rate of creatine phosphate resynthesis during the recovery periods. This increased rate of resynthesis resulted in the PCr content of the muscle being greater at the start of each subsequent sprint.

These improvements, however, may not be as pronounced in sprint running as found in cycling, as body mass (BM) has been shown to increase in some runners following acute creatine supplementation. This additional mass must be carried and propelled during running, attenuating some of the potential improvements in performance that might result from enhanced muscle power. Taken collectively, the results from the studies of the effects of recovery time on subsequent sprint performance combined with those of creatine supplementation strongly suggest that in order to maintain performance during sprinting, the muscle's energy status is more important than the direct effect of the H^+ on power output.

Carbohydrate availability

In a single 30-s sprint muscle glycogen drops by only 25–30%, suggesting that the stores are more than sufficient to fuel even a 400 m. However, in multiple sprints these muscle glycogen stores may become rapidly depleted. When subjects are required to perform a series of 10 6-s sprints with 30 s recovery on a cycle ergometer, the rate of glycogen use does not remain constant. Indeed, the rate of glycogen utilization is typically reduced by about 50% in the last compared to the first sprint, indicating that there is a progressive 'sparing' of glycogen and a concomitant increase in the contribution to energy provision by aerobic metabolism (Gaitanos *et al.* 1993).

Carbohydrate loading as used by endurance athletes (see Chapters 2 and 5) is not recommended for sprinters; the glycogen stores in the muscle are more than sufficient to fuel even the longest sprint. However, sprinters in training need to consume an adequate amount of carbohydrate (5–7 g·kg^{-1} BM) to replenish these stores on a daily basis.

Active vs. passive recovery

The effects of active recovery during repeated sprints have been investigated by Bogdanis *et al.* (1996). On two separate occasions these researchers examined subjects performing two 30-s sprints with 4 min recovery consisting of either an active or passive recovery.

The active recovery was low-intensity cycling at a work rate equivalent to about 40% of each athlete's $\dot{V}O_{2max}$. Active recovery resulted in a significantly higher mean power output in the second sprint compared with passive recovery, suggesting that the beneficial effects of active recovery were mediated by an increased blood flow to the previously exercised muscles. This enhanced blood flow would be expected to facilitate the restoration of the large changes in muscle metabolites through an increased supply of oxygen and a greater rate of removal of waste products. In particular, active recovery would increase blood lactate uptake and oxidation by the previously active, and inactive muscles. It is important, however, that the intensity of the active recovery is not so high as to cause further lactate accumulation in the muscle. Therefore, athletes should walk or jog gently between bouts of sprint running.

Environmental factors influencing sprint performance

Heat

It is generally accepted that performance of single sprint is enhanced when the active muscles are warmed by either an active warm-up or by artificially heating the muscles (e.g. by a water bath). In these situations the core temperature of the body is substantially below those levels at which performance would be impaired. However, is performance during activities requiring repeated short sprints affected by high thermal stresses resulting in elevated core temperatures?

Hot countries with high environmental stresses are frequently being chosen for international, Olympic and World Championships. For example, runners were regularly asked to perform in temperatures of 30–35 °C during both the Atlanta and Barcelona Olympics. At such temperatures there is no impairment in the performance of a single sprint. However, the capacity of the human body to dissipate the heat produced during exercise is compromised, reducing performance during prolonged submaximal exercise. It has been suggested that intermittent exercise may impose a greater thermal strain on the body than continuous exercise of an equivalent energy expenditure. One study has examined performance during intermittent high-intensity shuttle running in a hot (30 °C) and a moderate (20 °C) environment (Morris *et al.* 1996). The test utilized by these workers consisted of 15-m sprints interspersed by a three-phase sequence of walking, low-intensity jogging and high-intensity jogging, with each phase covering 60 m. The results of this study showed that the hot environment had a significant and detrimental effect on performance. The total distance covered before the subjects were too fatigued to continue, or forced to retire because of a rectal temperature greater than 39.5 °C, was less in the hot than for the moderate environment (8842 m vs. 11 201 m, respectively). Examination of each sprint performed revealed that sprint speed decreased with test time for all environmental conditions, with a tendency for the worst performance in the hot condition (Morris *et al.* 1996). If water was available for subjects to consume then, despite a rise in core temperature, performance did not differ greatly from the moderate condition. However, increasing the thermal stress by restricting fluid intake resulted in a marked decrement in sprint performance. It would appear therefore that in multiple sprint activities it is the attenuation of core temperature which is probably the determining factor affecting sprint performance.

Altitude

Air pressure, density and resistance decrease exponentially with altitude, being greatest at sea level. If air resistance was the only variable which affected running performance, then an improvement would be expected with increasing altitude. However, altitude causes not only a reduction in total air pressure but, more importantly, a reduction in the partial pressure of oxygen. This reduction in the partial pressure of oxygen occurs despite the chemical composition of the air remaining almost uniform. The reduced pressure of oxygen has, in turn, a direct effect on the saturation of blood with oxygen as it leaves the lungs. A reduced saturation thereby decreases the amount of oxygen being supplied to the working muscles per litre of cardiac output. This may attenuate performance during events placing a high demand on aerobic metabolism.

During the 1968 Mexico City Olympics (altitude 2300 m), performance in the sprint events was found to be the same or better than at sea level. However, in the middle distance races (e.g. 1500 m) performance was found to be impaired by about 3%, rising to about 8% for the longer distance events. Even at an altitude of only 1200 m performance in endurance events has been shown to be impaired.

Although aerobic metabolism during sprinting has been shown to be significant, most energy is supplied by the anaerobic power systems. Maximal anaerobic power appears to be unaffected by altitude. The potential slight loss in performance caused by attenuated aerobic metabolism appears to more than compensated for by reduced air resistance.

Although performance of single short sprints may benefit from altitude, the time taken to recover from these sprints is increased. Recovery between sprints is related to the maximum rate of aerobic metabolism, which is attenuated by altitude. This will, as a consequence, adversely affect sports requiring the individual to perform multiple sprints. Specific altitude training strategies for runners are discussed in more detail in Chapter 4.

Conclusions

The fibre composition of the propulsive muscles of sprinters has a marked influence on force generation and subsequent performance, with a high proportion of fast twitch muscle fibres being advantageous for a sprint runner. The fibre composition of the muscle is determined genetically with only limited scope for modification by training.

The performance of a single sprint appears to be influenced by the maximum rate at which energy can be supplied by anaerobic metabolism. Once the PCr stores in the muscle have been exhausted, which takes approximately 10 s, muscle tension is reduced by the inhibition of the cross-bridge cycle by the H^+ preventing the use of available ATP, while simultaneously reducing the rate of glycolysis. Both the rate of supply and utilization are affected by the composition of the muscle. Fast twitch fibres appear to have enhanced anaerobic enzyme activity leading towards optimization of the rate of glycolysis, while also having the ability to hydrolyse ATP at a very high rate, fuelling very rapid cross-bridge activity within the sarcomere. Consequently, these fibres are best able to generate large forces at high rates of muscle shortening to create most of the power required for sprinting.

During multiple sprints the maintenance of performance is influenced predominantly by the initial concentration and the subsequent restoration of muscle PCr stores. These stores are affected by the duration of the recovery period, with PCr resynthesis having a recovery half-time of approximately 50–60 s. This half-time is not a constant but is influenced by muscle pH, the availability of creatine and the aerobic fitness status of the athlete. If the recovery period is too short then sprint performance rapidly declines. This has direct implications for sprint training. If the quality of performance is to be maintained over a number of sprints then sufficient time is required between sprints for resynthesis of the PCr stores. Following a sprint during which the stores are depleted (i.e. longer than 10-s duration) it takes approximately 3 min for the stores to be replenished. Low-intensity active recovery between sprints appears to improve the rate of recovery, enabling sprint speed to be better maintained. The mode of recovery should use the previously exercised muscles and should not be of an intensity to cause further lactate accumulation.

Although sprints are predominantly fuelled by anaerobic metabolism, a significant contribution to the energy required for ATP resynthesis is derived from the aerobic energy systems, particularly in the longer duration sprints and in activities requiring repeated sprints. Runners with improved endurance fitness are best able to offset declines in sprint performance by increasing the contribution to energy provision from the aerobic systems during subsequent sprints.

References

Balsom, P.D., Ekblom, B., Soderlund, K., Sjodin, B. & Hultman, E. (1993) Creatine supplementation and dynamic high-intensity intermittent exercise. *Scandinavian Journal of Medicine and Science in Sports* **3**, 143–149.

Bogdanis, G.C., Nevill, M.E., Boobis, L.H. & Lakomy, H.K.A. (1994) Recovery of power output and muscle metabolites after 10 s and 20 s of maximal sprint exercise in man. *Clinical Science* **Suppl. 87**, 121–122.

Bogdanis, G.C., Nevill, M.E., Lakomy, H.K.A., Graham, C.M. & Louis, G. (1996) Effects of active recovery on power output during repeated maximal sprint cycling. *European Journal of Applied Physiology* **74**, 461–469.

Boobis, L., Williams, C. & Wootton, S. (1982) Human muscle metabolism during brief maximal exercise. *Journal of Physiology* **338**, 21–22.

Dowson, M.N., Nevill, M.E., Lakomy, H.K.A., Nevill, A.M. & Hazeldine, R.J. (1998) Modeling the relationship between isokinetic muscle strength and sprint running performance. *Journal of Sports Sciences* **16**, 257–265.

Esbjornsson, M., Sylven, C., Holm, I. & Jansson, E. (1993) Fast twitch fibres may predict anaerobic performance in both females and males. *International Journal of Sports Medicine* **14**, 257–263.

Fukunaga, T., Matsuo, A., Yuasa, K., Fujimatsu, H. & Asahina, K. (1978) Mechanical power output in running. *Biomechanics* VI-B, 17–22.

Gaitanos, G.C., Williams, C., Boobis, L. & Brooks, S. (1993) Human muscle metabolism during intermittent maximal exercise. *Journal of Applied Physiology* **75**, 712–719.

Holmyard, D., Cheetham, M.E., Lakomy, H. & Williams, C. (1988) Effect of recovery duration on performance during multiple sprint treadmill sprints. *Proceedings of the First World Congress of Science and Football* **13**, 134–142.

Katz, A., Sahlin, K. & Henriksson, J. (1986) Muscle ATP turnover rate during isometric contraction in humans. *Journal of Applied Physiology* **60**, 1839–1842.

Koshla, T. (1978) Standards of age, height and weight in Olympic running events for men. *British Journal of Sports Medicine* **12**, 97–101.

Koshla, T. & McBroome, V.C. (1984) *The Physique of Female Olympic Finalists*, pp. 1–13. Welsh School of Medicine, Cardiff, Wales.

Lakomy, H.K. (1984) An ergometer for measuring the power generated during sprinting. *Journal of Physiology* **354**, 33.

Lakomy, H.K. (1986) Measurement of work and power output generated on friction-loaded cycle ergometers. *Ergonomics* **29**, 509–514.

McCartney, N., Heigenhauser, G.J.F. & Jones, N.L. (1983) Power output and fatigue of human muscle in maximal cycling exercise. *Journal of Applied Physiology* **55**, 218–224.

Morris, J.G., Nevill, M.E., Lakomy, H.K.A., Nicholas, C. & Williams, C. (1996) Effect of a hot environment on performance of prolonged intermittent, high intensity shuttle running. *Journal of Sports Sciences* **14**, 94.

Nevill, M.E., Boobis, L.H., Brooks, S. & Williams, C. (1989) Effect of training on muscle metabolism during treadmill sprinting. *Journal of Applied Physiology* **67**, 2376–2382.

Recommended reading

Williams, C. & Gandy, G. (1994) Physiology and nutrition for sprinting. In: *Perspectives in Exercise Science and Sports Medicine* Vol. 7. *Physiology and Nutrition for Competitive Sport* (eds D.R. Lamb, H.G. Knuttgen & R. Murray), pp. 55–98. Cooper Publishing Group, Carmel, Indiana.

Chapter 2

Physiology and biochemistry

of middle distance and

long distance running

The closing years of this century have seen enormous improvements in the standard of middle distance running at world level, as evidenced by dramatic reductions in the world records (Table 2.1). However, several long distance records (the marathon distance, for example) have, until very recently, been relatively static, with little rate of improvement. In many countries the standard of competition at regional and national level has actually declined over the same period. It is interesting to speculate on the social and other changes that might account for these trends, but it is clear that the projected limit to human performance at these events has not yet been reached. Further improvements will occur, although a point must come when no additional progress will be possible. The physiology of the elite runner in middle distance and distance events lies at the extreme of the human gene pool and gives some insight as to the factors that might ultimately limit performance.

For the purposes of this chapter, running events at all distances from 800 m upwards will be considered. Events from 800 to 5000 m are usually classified as 'middle distance' and events at 10 000 m or longer as 'distance' races. Based on the physiological demands of the events, the runners' distinction between middle distance and long distance is a realistic one: the requirements for successful performance at the marathon distance are quite different from those at 800 m. Races at distances longer that the marathon (42.2 km, or 26.2 miles) are commonly termed 'ultradistance'. In recent years, popular participation in marathon races has declined, and many of the big city marathons have been largely replaced by events at distances of 10 km or at the half-marathon distance. Among serious athletes, there has been a growing interest in ultra-distance races, especially over 100 km or 24 h. Although these races remain very much

Table 2.1 World record performances for men and women at distances from 800 m to 100 km in 1978 and 1998. All performances are track records, except for the marathon distance (42.2 km)

	Men		Women	
Distance (km)	1978	1998	1978	1998
0.8	1:43.40	1:41.11	1:54.90	1:53.28
1.5	3:32.2	3:26.00	3:56.00	3:50.46
1.6	3:49.4	3:44.39	4:23.8	4:12.56
2	4:51.4	4:47.88	–	5:25.36
3	7:32.1	7:20.67	8:27.2	8:06.11
5	13:08.4	12:39.36	15:08.8	14:28.09
10	27:22.5	26:22.75	33:34.2	29:31.78
42.2	2:08:34	2:06:50	2:34:47	2:20:47
50		2:43:38		3:08:39
100	6:10:20	6:10:20		7:00:48

minority events with a select band of participants, they do raise some interesting and unique physiological problems.

Energy demands of middle and long distance running

Those runners who can sustain a higher average speed over the entire distance of a race than anyone has previously achieved break world records. This requires a high rate of energy production to be sustained throughout a race. In competition, and especially in major championship events, the picture is somewhat complicated by tactical rather than physiological considerations, and the runner who wins is often the one who is capable of a short burst of high-intensity effort in the closing stages of the race. Variations in environmental conditions and, at least in road and cross-country races, in the surface and elevation, as well as variations in pace throughout the race, will lead to a fluctuating energy demand.

The energy for muscle contraction comes from the breakdown of adenosine triphosphate (ATP) and muscular work can be sustained only if the ATP concentration in the cell is maintained: this means that the rate of ATP resynthesis must equal the rate of ATP hydrolysis. At all distances, the energy for ATP resynthesis will be provided from a combination of aerobic

Table 2.2 The approximate contributions of anaerobic and aerobic energy metabolism to the total energy cost of maximum performance at different durations of exercise. Times shown are the current (November 1999) men's world records at these distances

Distance	Time	Aerobic energy (%)	Anaerobic energy (%)
100 m	0:09.79	10	90
400 m	0:43.29	30	70
800 m	1:41.11	60	40
1500 m	3:26.00	80	20
5000 m	12:39.36	95	5
10 000 m	26:22.75	97	3
42.2 km	2:05.42	> 99	< 1

and anaerobic sources; at the shorter race distances, the contribution of anaerobic metabolism will be substantial (see Chapter 1), but this energy source will have little part to play in the long distance events (Table 2.2). Anaerobic energy metabolism allows high rates of power output to fuel maximal effort. However, the capacity of the anaerobic power system (the total amount of energy that can be produced) is relatively small. The maximum rate of energy supplied by aerobic metabolism is much less than the anaerobic system and is limited by the maximum rate of oxidative metabolism (normally expressed as the maximum oxygen uptake, $\dot{V}O_{2max}$). In middle distance running, the rate of energy expenditure is much greater than the rate at which oxidative metabolism can supply energy, and a high capacity for anaerobic metabolism is essential for successful performance. At the longer distances, an effective aerobic power system is the major prerequisite for top performance.

Anaerobic power and capacity

Anaerobic ATP formation is necessary to supplement oxidative metabolism in the first few minutes of exercise until oxygen delivery increases to meet the demand, and also where the power output demands a rate of energy utilization greater than that which can be met by oxidative metabolism alone (see Chapter 1). From measurements of the total energy cost of work and the amount of oxygen consumed ($\dot{V}O_2$), it is possible to calculate the relative contribution of anaerobic

metabolism to the total energy demand to be about 20% in a maximum effort of 4 min duration, decreasing to less than 1% in maximal exercise lasting for 2 h (Table 2.2).

The energy supplied by anaerobic metabolism can be conveniently expressed in terms of the equivalent oxygen consumption. The anaerobic capacity ranges from 52 ml·kg⁻¹ in untrained individuals up to 90 ml·kg⁻¹ in sprinters, figures that correspond to just over 1 min at the maximum rate of energy production via aerobic metabolism (Medbo *et al.* 1988). Interestingly, it has been shown that at least 2 min of exercise are necessary to maximally tax the anaerobic capacity; in longer duration exercise, lasting about 9 min or more, there is no further change in the total contribution of anaerobic metabolism (Medbo *et al.* 1988).

To put these values in context it has been estimated that the oxygen cost of running 1609 m (1 mile) in a time of 4 min (an average speed of 6.67 m·s⁻¹) is about 84 ml·kg⁻¹·min⁻¹, which equates to a total oxygen cost of 23.5 l for a 70-kg runner (Snell 1990). Using such values, a 70-kg runner with a $\dot{V}O_{2max}$ of 70 ml·kg⁻¹·min⁻¹ would incur an oxygen deficit of *c.* 4.9 l. To break the current world record of 3 min 44.39 s would require an oxygen cost of *c.* 105 ml·kg⁻¹·min⁻¹; this clearly requires that both the anaerobic and aerobic systems are at the upper limits of their capacity. In addition, an economical running style that can decrease the energy cost of running would be a major benefit.

In events of longer duration, the contribution of anaerobic metabolism to energy production declines, and the requirement for a high anaerobic capacity is correspondingly less important. Highly trained elite runners can race 5000 m at an intensity at or close to their $\dot{V}O_{2max}$, and the substantial oxygen deficit incurred in the first few minutes will persist or even increase as the race progresses. Even at longer distances, anaerobic energy production will occur at intermediate points in a race if the pace is increased or during bouts of uphill running. Some anaerobic effort is also normally involved in the closing stages during a sprint finish. Most world class male 10 000-m runners are capable of running 1609 m (1 mile) in rather less than 4 min.

The anaerobic power that can be produced by endurance runners in standardized laboratory tests is, as might be expected, rather low compared with that of trained sprint athletes. Marathon runners demonstrate low isometric strength of the quadriceps muscles relative to sprinters and even tend to have less muscle strength than healthy but untrained individuals. These observations are perhaps unsurprising in view of the generally smaller muscle mass of the distance runners and of the high proportion of type I fibres present in their muscles. However, they may also reflect the training patterns of these athletes (see Chapter 4).

Aerobic power

As the duration of running events increases, so does the proportion of the total energy demand that must be met by oxidative metabolism. Running speed declines as the competition distance increases but, based on current world records, it is apparent that the decrease in speed, and hence in oxygen demand, is rather gradual with increasing duration of effort (Fig. 2.1).

Few successful male runners have failed to record $\dot{V}_{O_{2max}}$ values of at least 70 ml·kg^{-1}·min^{-1}, compared with values of 40–45 ml·kg^{-1}·min^{-1} for sedentary individuals. Values recorded for elite female distance runners are only slightly less than those of males. There have been several reports of individual $\dot{V}_{O_{2max}}$ values of 80–85 ml·kg^{-1}·min^{-1}, and it is notable that such exceptionally high values are more common in middle distance than in long distance athletes. The highest reported value (recorded in a reputable laboratory) for a female runner appears to be that of Grete Waitz of Norway, who recorded 73.3 ml·kg^{-1}·min^{-1} and had a best marathon time of 2:25:29. In a large group of elite American female distance runners, including specialists at both middle and long distance events, $\dot{V}_{O_{2max}}$ values ranging from 61 to 73 ml·kg^{-1}·min^{-1} (with a mean value of 68.0 ml·kg^{-1}·min^{-1} for the middle distance runners and 66.4 ml·kg^{-1}·min^{-1} for the long distance specialists) have been reported (Pate *et al.* 1987). Although a large part of the difference in $\dot{V}_{O_{2max}}$ values between male and female runners can be accounted for by differences in body fat content, even when values are expressed relative to lean body mass, the values obtained by women are still less than those of the best men.

When comparisons are made within groups of runners of widely different levels of performance, a good

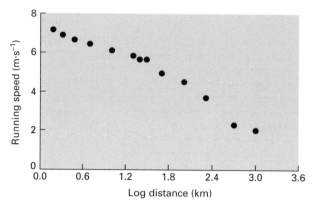

Fig. 2.1 Running speed declines with distance for all athletes. This is demonstrated by an examination of the current world records at different distances. The shape of the curve, however, is not the same for an individual as it is for these composite data; the decline in the maximum sustainable speed with increasing distance will be more pronounced for the middle distance runner than for the ultra-marathon runner.

relationship between running performance and an athlete's $\dot{V}_{O_{2max}}$ is apparent. This is true for middle distance events as well as for long distance events (see Maughan 1994). The relationship between finishing time in a marathon race and $\dot{V}_{O_{2max}}$ measured within a few weeks of a race is shown in Fig. 2.2.

Although there is a reasonably good relationship between $\dot{V}_{O_{2max}}$ and average marathon speed, no such relationship is seen if individuals of similar performance level are compared. This suggests that, although a high capacity for oxidative metabolism is necessary for success in distance running, it does not, in itself, distinguish the elite performer. It is not unusual to find male club athletes who can achieve $\dot{V}_{O_{2max}}$ values in excess of 75 ml·kg^{-1}·min^{-1} in spite of their relatively modest performances. Similarly, much has been made of the fact that some exceptional runners have failed to produce outstanding results in the laboratory. A runner whose best marathon performance was 2:08:33 was found to have a $\dot{V}_{O_{2max}}$ of 'only' 70 ml·kg^{-1}·min^{-1} while a 2:10 marathon runner was recently reported to have attained a $\dot{V}_{O_{2max}}$ of just 67 ml·kg^{-1}·min^{-1}. Similarly modest values have been recorded for some elite middle distance runners: for example, a value of 72 ml·kg^{-1}·min^{-1} was reported for Peter Snell whose best mile time was 3 min 54.5 s, compared with 84.4 ml·kg^{-1}·min^{-1} for Steve Prefontaine

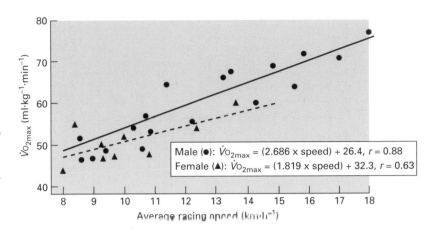

Fig. 2.2 The relationship between maximum oxygen uptake achieved in a laboratory treadmill running test and performance in male and female competitors in a marathon (42.2 km) race. Performance is expressed as the average running speed for the complete distance. All subjects took part in the same race and all measurements were made within 2 weeks of the completion of the race. Reproduced with permission from Maughan and Leiper (1983).

whose best mile performance was almost identical (3 min 54.6 s). Although there have been dramatic improvements in world middle distance records over recent years, laboratory measurements made on Don Lash, whose best mile time of 4 min 7.2 s in 1937 was achieved with an oxygen uptake of 81.5 ml·kg^{-1}·min^{-1}, suggest that improvements in running records cannot be attributed simply to greater aerobic power.

Before looking for a physiological explanation for these seemingly anomalous observations, it should be remembered that, in many of these studies, measurements were made at a time when the runners who were tested were not at their peak racing fitness. The information is not usually given, but it is apparent that, in some cases, the laboratory test was separated by a period of months or even years from the time when the runner's best performance, to which the laboratory tests are related, was achieved. In addition, the exercise protocol in some cases involved horizontal running at increasing velocities, which is likely to result in termination of the test before a true $\dot{V}O_{2max}$ is reached.

Fractional utilization of aerobic capacity

In middle distance events, runners are working at intensities close to or above $\dot{V}O_{2max}$. Trained runners reach their maximum rate of oxygen consumption after about 3 min of exercise and can sustain 100% of $\dot{V}O_{2max}$ for about 7 min, 85–90% for 60 min and 80–85% for 120 min (Peronnet & Thibault 1989). In the longer events, where the energy demand is met almost entirely by aerobic metabolism, runners with

a high $\dot{V}O_{2max}$ can meet the oxygen requirement by employing a relatively low fraction of their maximum. Conversely, runners who have a lower $\dot{V}O_{2max}$ have to work at a relatively higher intensity to run at the same speed. Part of the apparent lack of a close association between $\dot{V}O_{2max}$ and performance in long distance races may be accounted for by differences between individuals in the fraction of $\dot{V}O_{2max}$ that can be sustained for the duration of a race. Although a good relationship between marathon running performance and the fraction of $\dot{V}O_{2max}$ that can be sustained for the duration of the race is seen when runners of widely different levels of ability are compared (Fig. 2.3), there is generally no such relationship seen when homogeneous groups are compared.

The general trend (Fig. 2.3) does, however, suggest that the fastest runners are able to run at a high fraction of $\dot{V}O_{2max}$ over any given distance. This is hardly surprising, as the fraction of $\dot{V}O_{2max}$ that can be maintained is more closely related to time than to distance, and the faster runners take less time to cover any given distance (Maughan 1990). For any individual, however, the fraction of $\dot{V}O_{2max}$ that can be sustained decreases with the distance. One early study (Davies & Thompson 1979) found that a group of highly trained marathon runners utilized 94% of their $\dot{V}O_{2max}$ over 5 km (15 min 49 s), 82% over 42.2 km (2:31) and 67% over 84.4 km (5:58). One of the major effects of endurance training sustained over a period of many years is to increase the ability to utilize a large fraction of $\dot{V}O_{2max}$ for prolonged periods, and hence substantial improvements in racing performance can be achieved without any significant change in $\dot{V}O_{2max}$.

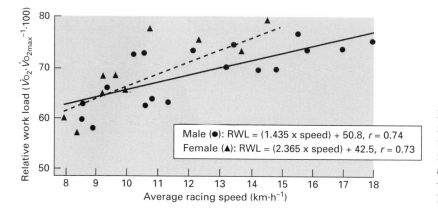

Fig. 2.3 The relationship between marathon performance and fractional utilization of maximum oxygen uptake in the same group of marathon runners as presented in Fig. 2.2. Reproduced with permission from Maughan and Leiper (1983).

Biomechanics and running economy

It requires no sophisticated laboratory analysis to distinguish between the elite runner and the jogger. Even the untrained eye can see the difference between the fluent running action of the best distance runners and that of the more modest performer. There are some prominent exceptions to this generalization, but they are few.

An individual's running style is partly an innate characteristic but is also the result of a modification of this style by training. Comparisons of the running economy (measured as the energy cost of running at a fixed submaximal speed) of identical and non-identical twin brothers have indicated that there is no genetic component to running economy. There is some evidence that training status is an important determinant of running economy, and runners covering long weekly training distances can generally run at a variety of speeds with a lower $\dot{V}O_2$ than runners who do less training. This suggests that there may be advantages to a high training volume, although most of the improvements in performance are normally associated with high-intensity training (see Chapter 4). As might be expected, running economy is a more important determinant of success at long rather than at the shorter distances. A number of studies have shown that elite distance runners use 5–10% less oxygen than either non-elite runners or middle distance runners (see Maughan 1994).

Even among elite runners, however, there may be large differences in the oxygen cost of running. Some studies have shown that the oxygen cost of running at a given speed is a good predictor of performance, but there are many studies that have found no such relationship. In spite of this conflict, a review of published data shows that the lowest oxygen uptake values at fixed running speeds have been recorded by the world's best distance runners (Sjodin & Svedenhag 1985), suggesting that running economy is a major factor for successful distance running performance. It may be important for the middle distance runner to be able to run fast; as long ago as 1926, it was shown that the oxygen cost of running at a fixed submaximal speed was inversely related to the best time achieved for 400 m. More recently, it has been shown that the fastest speed that can be sustained for 5 s on a treadmill is very closely related ($r = 0.89$) to the best time over 5000 m (Scott & Houmard 1994).

There have been several attempts to identify factors which might account for the differences in running economy which exist among runners. It seems that many different factors, including stride length and frequency, and the vertical oscillation with each stride, made a small contribution to the differences which exist between individuals. It is well recognized that the oxygen cost of running at a constant speed increases over time during endurance events, indicating a decrease in running economy. Part of the increase in $\dot{V}O_2$ is a result of a gradual change in substrate utilization by the muscles; fat oxidation provides only 20.2 kJ·l⁻¹ (4.8 kcal·l⁻¹) of oxygen compared with the higher energy yield (21.059 kJ·l⁻¹ or 5.014 kcal·l⁻¹) available when carbohydrate is oxidized. This cannot be the only reason, however, as running economy deteriorates to the same extent whether or not carbohydrate is supplied during exercise. The fatigued runner is generally less well coordinated, and there may be changes in the muscle recruitment pattern as fatigue develops that are responsible for the reduced efficiency.

Characteristics of elite runners

Physical characteristics

Age

Athletic performance deteriorates with age but the age at which optimum performance can be expected to occur in different events is not clear. Most elite distance runners record their best performances between the ages of 20 and 30 years, and a study of the ages of medal winners at major championships and of world record holders tends to confirm this. Table 2.3 shows the ages of the top ranked men and women in the world at various race distances for 1997.

There is a general trend for sprinters to be younger than distance runners, and most runners find that their preferred race distance increases as they grow older. An examination of world age bests at different race distances suggests that running performance deteriorates in both sprint and long distance events, but that the rate of decrease in sprinting ability is greater than that in endurance capacity. These data may, of course, be invalid because of a tendency for sprint athletes to retire completely from the sport when their performances begin to decline.

As with all generalizations, there are many exceptions. Several of the top male sprinters at the 1992 Barcelona Olympics, including the 100 m gold

medallist (Linford Christie, UK), were considerably older than all of the medallists in the marathon. Two of the top 10 ranked women 100-m runners in 1997 were over the age of 30 years, and the third fastest woman was a 37-year-old. In spite of the regulations, which prevent young athletes from running marathons in some countries, some young athletes can achieve outstanding performances.

Body composition

There are substantial differences in many of the physical characteristics of sprinters and long distance runners, but elite distance runners come in a variety of shapes and sizes, and there are perhaps too many exceptions to make all but the broadest generalizations. The one outstanding anthropometric characteristic of successful competitors in all distance running events is a low body fat content. Estimates of the body composition in 114 male runners at the 1968 US Olympic Trial race yielded an average fat content of 7.5% of body mass, less than half that of a physically active but not highly trained group (Costill *et al.* 1970). The low body fat content of female distance runners is particularly striking, and values of less than 12–14% are commonly reported among elite performers. In a study of a population of runners who were rather heterogeneous with respect to their training status and athletic ability, a significant relationship between body composition and the best time that could be achieved over a distance of 3208 m (2 miles) has been observed (Housh *et al.* 1986). This relationship may, at least in part, be explained by an association between the amount of training carried out and the body composition: body fat content tends to decrease as the volume of training increases (Fig. 2.4).

Fat is an important fuel for the working muscles in distance running and has a number of other important metabolic and hormonal roles, but excess body fat serves no useful function and adds to the mass that a runner must carry, thus increasing the energy cost of running. A 60-kg runner with 5% body fat will have about 3 kg of fat, while a 55-kg female runner with 15% body fat will have more than 8 kg of body fat. Non-elite runners will commonly have up to twice this amount of body fat. Although there may be short-term performance gains in reducing the body fat to

Table 2.3 The mean age (±SD) in years of the top 10 performers in the world at selected distances for 1997

Distance	Men	Women
100 m	25.4 (3.8)	26.1 (5.1)
1500 m	26.8 (3.5)	21.4 (3.9)
10 000 m	25.5 (4.3)	22.5 (3.7)
Marathon	29.2 (3.3)	27.2 (4.4)

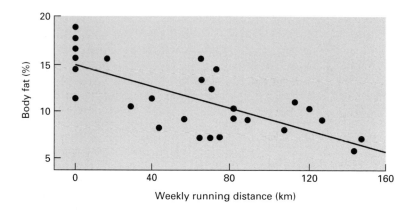

Fig. 2.4 Body fat content estimated in a group of male runners who were in a steady-state with respect to training load and body composition, and in a group of weight-stable sedentary control subjects. The runners had all been training for at least 2 years and had completed the same weekly training distance without any change in body weight for at least 10 weeks prior to the time of measurement. One of the effects of a high training load is to maintain a low body fat content.

very low levels, there are adverse effects on health and on the capacity to train intensively in the longer term, especially in female runners, where a low body fat content and a high training load may lead to menstrual irregularities.

Muscle fibre composition and metabolic profile

Chapter 1 described the two main types of muscle fibres. Slow twitch fibres (also known as type I fibres) contract relatively slowly, and are resistant to fatigue, relying mainly on aerobic metabolism for energy supply. Fast twitch (type II) fibres shorten at a higher speed and can generate high power outputs because of their greater capacity for anaerobic energy metabolism. The fast twitch fibres can be further subdivided into type IIa fibres which have a high aerobic capacity, and type IIb fibres which have a low aerobic capacity. Slow twitch fibres predominate in the muscles of elite endurance runners, while elite sprinters have muscles that consist mostly of fast twitch fibres (see Chapter 1), with approximately equal numbers of type I and II fibres in the leg muscles of middle distance runners (Saltin *et al.* 1977). In non-elite runners performing at lower levels of competition, however, a wide spread of fibre compositions will be observed at any distance. As well as differences in the numbers of the different fibre types, the fibres may be different sizes. The cross-sectional area of the type II fibres of sprinters may be almost twice as great as that of their type I fibres, but size differences between fibre types are much less apparent in marathon runners.

The muscles of endurance-trained individuals, or at least those muscles which have been trained, have a high capacity for oxidative metabolism; the mitochondrial density is high and the activity of the enzymes involved in oxidation of carbohydrate, and more especially of fat, is correspondingly high. These muscles also have a dense capillary network, allowing an increased blood flow to the muscle and an increased capillary transit time. The major significance of the local adaptations within the muscle may be an increased capacity for the use of fat as a fuel, leading to a slower rate of depletion of the limited muscle glycogen stores: at the same running speed, the trained distance runner has a greater rate of fat oxidation. This is partly because of the increased delivery of bloodborne free fatty acids because of the increased capillary supply of the muscle, and partly to the enhanced capacity of the muscle to oxidize fat.

Exercise intensity is a major factor influencing the adaptive response of muscle and of the different fibre types. This reflects the use of the different fibres during running. During slow running, only the type I fibres are active; the type II fibres will only be used in the later stages of prolonged slow runs when the type I fibres become fatigued. However, as running speed increases, the type IIa fibres begin to be recruited, and at very high speeds all of the fibres are active. Long slow distance running will not therefore cause training adaptations in the fibres that are not recruited, but fast interval training sessions will train all of the muscle fibres. Training volume is generally proportional to racing distance, and intensity is inversely related to volume (see Chapter 4), so the higher training intensities of runners competing at distances of 800 m up to 5000 m will result in greater adaptations of the type II fibres. High-speed running, eliciting more than 80% of

$\dot{V}O_{2max}$ appears to be necessary to produce a training response in the type IIb fibres. Marathon runners whose training consists primarily of long slow runs will seldom reach this intensity in training, and it is perhaps unsurprising that, even among long distance runners, there has been a trend towards a reduction in training volume and an increase in intensity in recent years (see Chapter 4).

The high oxidative capacity of the muscles of the elite endurance athlete is, in part, a reflection of the high proportion of type I fibres present. Because the proportions of the different fibre types in the muscle are genetically determined, there is a large genetic component to success at the highest level. The activity of enzymes involved in oxidative metabolism is, however, generally high in both of the major fibre types in highly trained middle and long distance runners, reflecting an adaptation to the training programme. The muscles have a great capacity for adaptation to specific training stimuli, and the oxidative capacity of the type II fibres of the highly trained endurance athlete may exceed that of the type I fibres of the sedentary individual. There are still, however, distinct fibre types present in the trained muscle, and the oxidative capacity of type II fibres does not exceed that of type I fibres from the same individual. The time course of adaptation of the muscles to training and detraining is different from that of the observed changes in $\dot{V}O_{2max}$, and the magnitude of the responses is quite different: enzyme activity changes rapidly in response to changes in the training load, and the changes are rather large relative to the changes in $\dot{V}O_{2max}$ (Henriksson & Hickner 1992).

Gender

Current world record performances for men and women at a variety of distances have been compared in Table 2.1. The ratio of the women's to the men's performances is relatively constant at about 90% across a wide range of distances (this ratio is 89% at 1500 m and 88% at 100 km). The relatively poorer performances of women at some distances probably reflects the comparatively short history of women's participation in these events. Some of the factors which may account for performance differences between men and women are identified in Table 2.4.

Table 2.4 Some of the factors which may account for performance differences between male and female runners

Variable	Performance parameter
Muscle mass	Force production
	Peak power output
Body composition	Oxygen cost of running
Heart size	Maximum oxygen uptake
Haemoglobin concentration	Maximum oxygen uptake
Muscle enzyme activity	Relative use of fat and carbohydrate as fuels
Biomechanical differences	Running economy

Peak power output of women is generally lower than that of men, reflecting in part the lower muscle mass, as muscle strength per unit of muscle mass is generally similar in men and women. Female athletes generally achieve lower $\dot{V}O_{2max}$ values than those of men competing in the same events. Part of this difference is a consequence of the higher body fat content of women, but the differences persist even after correction for body mass and body fat content. A number of other factors contribute to the lower $\dot{V}O_{2max}$ of women. These include a lower maximum cardiac output and, because maximum heart rates are similar, this reflects a smaller stroke volume. Differences in cardiac size between trained men and women can account for about 70% of the difference in $\dot{V}O_{2max}$. Blood haemoglobin concentration is generally lower in women than in men and this may also have some significance for oxygen transport. Hard endurance training tends to lower the circulating haemoglobin concentration and anaemia may be a problem for some runners; the low haemoglobin concentration of highly trained endurance athletes, whether male or female, is, however, most commonly a pseudo-anaemia resulting from a disproportionate expansion of the plasma volume. The potentially adverse effects of a low haemoglobin concentration may be offset, at least in part, by the raised 2,3-diphosphoglycerate (DPG) content of red blood cells seen in endurance-trained women.

Muscle fibre distribution shows a normal distribution in both male and female runners, with no gender difference in the relative proportions of the major fibre types present. There have been suggestions of an increased reliance on fat as a metabolic fuel during exercise in women, leading to a sparing of glycogen, but there are conflicting reports in the literature (see Maughan 1990 for a review of these studies).

Potential limitations to middle and long distance running performance

Although there is clearly a limit to the performance of all runners, it is unlikely that any single factor limits the performance of all individuals in all situations. None the less, several clues as to the possible limitations to performance in middle and long distance running are readily apparent from the study of the characteristics of elite performers. Other information comes from measurements made during competition or in the laboratory, but the evidence is inevitably circumstantial at best, and the limitations of our knowledge must be recognized.

Cardiovascular and pulmonary function

The primary requirement for successful performance in middle distance events is the ability to sustain a high power output for short periods of time, whereas the challenge facing the long distance runner is that of maintaining a submaximal effort over prolonged periods. For the middle distance runner, a high $\dot{V}_{O_{2max}}$ is therefore a prerequisite, whereas the long distance runner can compensate to some degree for a lower $\dot{V}_{O_{2max}}$ by the ability to sustain a high fraction of aerobic power for prolonged periods.

The various factors which might limit $\dot{V}_{O_{2max}}$ have been reviewed elsewhere (Maughan 1992), and there has been considerable debate as to where the limitation(s) to $\dot{V}_{O_{2max}}$ reside. Endurance-trained individuals have a highly developed cardiovascular system, and their muscles also have a high capacity for oxidative metabolism. The balance of the available evidence suggests that, where a large muscle mass is involved, as in running, oxygen utilization is limited by the rate at which it can be delivered to the working muscles rather than by the capacity of those muscles to utilize oxygen. There remain, however, several potential limitations to oxygen delivery.

Until recently it was generally considered that there was no limitation to oxygen uptake imposed by the lungs. There were, however, some reports suggesting that the elite athlete may be limited by ventilation. One study (Martin *et al.* 1985) reported that elite male distance runners achieved ventilation rates during exercise that approached their voluntary ventilatory limits, and a number of more recent reports have provided more convincing evidence by demonstrating arterial desaturation during hard exercise in endurance-trained subjects. The implication of these observations is that there may be a pulmonary limitation to oxygen transport. In as many as 50% of elite distance runners, the arterial oxygen saturation may fall during sea level exercise at running intensities close to $\dot{V}_{O_{2max}}$. The oxygen content of the blood may fall in exercise at intensities close to maximum because of a mismatch between perfusion of the vascular bed and local diffusion capacity. When the cardiac output is very high, pulmonary capillary transit time may be too short to allow complete equilibration to occur. The fact that desaturation occurs in athletes rather than in sedentary individuals may be a consequence of the small changes in lung function that occur with most types of training. Elite distance runners can achieve a cardiac output 2–3 times greater than that of sedentary individuals, but the differences in maximum ventilatory function and pulmonary diffusion capacity are small. There are, however, reports which suggest that specific training of the lungs may improve endurance performance in both trained and untrained individuals. Distance runners should perhaps give some thought to efforts to improve functional lung capacity. Not all runners show arterial desaturation during high intensity exercise, but those who do will be particularly liable to suffer decrements in performance during events held at altitude.

An individual's $\dot{V}_{O_{2max}}$ is closely related to the maximum cardiac output that can be attained. The maximum heart rate is little influenced by training status and tends, if anything, to decrease, so it is clear that stroke volume is a major determinant of $\dot{V}_{O_{2max}}$ and hence of distance running performance. Blood volume and the circulating haemoglobin concentration also have an influence on $\dot{V}_{O_{2max}}$, and the practice of removal and subsequent reinfusion of whole blood or red blood cells has been employed by athletes to improve performance, with apparent success. For example, it has been shown that a plasma volume expander can increase the circulating volume by about 4% and elevate $\dot{V}O_{2max}$ by a similar amount; larger increases are not effective, presumably because of the haemodilution that results (Coyle *et al.* 1990). In view of these observations and of the importance of the oxygen-carrying capacity of the blood for oxygen transport, the decrease in circulating haemoglobin concentration which commonly occurs in trained athletes seems surprising. This condition, often referred to as sports anaemia, is not a true anaemia, however, as the total red cell mass is unchanged or even increased, but is the result of a disproportionate increase in the plasma volume in response to the training stimulus. Altitude training (see Chapter 4), red blood cell transfusions, and the use of erythropoietin (EPO) to stimulate the formation of new red blood cells are all strategies that have been used in sport to try to increase the oxygen carrying capacity of the blood (for review see Eichner 1992).

Energy metabolism

The relative contributions of anaerobic and aerobic metabolism to energy production in events over different distances have been discussed earlier in this chapter. The primary factor influencing the metabolic response to running is the intensity; the higher the intensity, the greater the energy demand and the greater the proportion of the total energy turnover that is met by carbohydrate metabolism. When the running speed elicits close to 95% of an athlete's $\dot{V}O_{2max}$, the contribution of fat oxidation to energy metabolism is negligible. Using an estimate of 5.9 l·min⁻¹ as the oxygen cost of a 70-kg runner running at 4 min a mile pace, and assuming that the entire energy demand could be met by oxidation of muscle glycogen (Snell 1990), it can be calculated that the rate of carbohydrate oxidation necessary to meet this rate of energy expenditure would be 7.5 g·min⁻¹. Assuming, however, that the energy supply can be met entirely by anaerobic glycolysis, the rate of carbohydrate degradation would be approximately 100 g·min⁻¹. For a runner with a $\dot{V}O_{2max}$ of 70 ml·kg⁻¹·min⁻¹, who can use 75% of that value in the first minute of a race and 100% thereafter, and ignoring the contribution of creatine phosphate hydrolysis, the total carbohydrate degradation during a 1609-m (1-mile) race would be

about 110 g. Of this amount some 85 g would be converted to lactate which, if distributed equally throughout 85% of the body water space, would reach a concentration of just over 26 mmol·l⁻¹. This latter value is very close to those observed during experimental conditions, and is close to the highest values ever recorded.

These rough calculations show that the amount of muscle glycogen used is small relative to the whole body glycogen store, and that substrate availability should not be limiting in events over this distance. There are, however, suggestions that the availability of muscle glycogen may limit the performance of events of this duration (Maughan & Greenhall 1991), perhaps because of depletion in specific muscle fibre pools. The implications of lactate accumulation for acid–base status and fatigue are discussed below.

At submaximal exercise intensities the contribution of fat oxidation to energy production increases with time, but the contribution of fat to energy metabolism is likely to be insignificant at distances of less than 10 km run at race pace. Even at the marathon distance, where the energy demand can be met almost entirely by aerobic metabolism, the total amount of fat oxidized is small; if fat was the only fuel used the total amount oxidized in a race would be no more than about 300 g. In contrast, if carbohydrate was the only fuel used the total would be about 700 g, an amount that is in excess of the amount that is normally stored in the working muscles and liver. Carbohydrate availability is widely recognized as a potential limitation to long distance running performance, and carbohydrate ingestion during distance running is effective in improving performance (see Chapter 5).

Disturbances in acid–base status

Anaerobic glycolysis meets a large part of the energy demand in middle distance races but is relatively unimportant in long distance events. When the rate of carbohydrate breakdown by the glycolytic enzymes in the cytoplasm exceeds the rate at which the pyruvate produced can be converted to carbon dioxide and water in the mitochondria, conversion of some of the pyruvate to lactate allows glycolysis to continue. Some of the hydrogen ions that are produced along with the lactate are buffered by the intracellular buffers (primarily proteins) and some diffuse into the extracellular space where further buffering occurs (primarily by bicarbonate). The buffering, however, is incomplete, and the pH of the intracellular and extracellular spaces will fall when there is significant lactate accumulation.

There are several possible mechanisms by which a fall in pH may result in fatigue. It must be emphasized, however, that anaerobic glycolysis does allow a high rate of ATP production to be maintained; reductions in the glycolytic rate, if not compensated for by other sources of energy production, would have the effect of reducing exercise capacity. Increasing buffering capacity, on the other hand, might be expected to improve performance if the fall in pH is indeed limiting. In simulated competition over distances of 800 and 1500 m, the ingestion of sodium bicarbonate in the prerace period has been shown to improve performance by 3–5 s. However, these studies used club level runners and equivalent improvements are unlikely to occur with elite runners. It should also be noted that there is some risk of acute gastrointestinal distress when the large doses of bicarbonate necessary to produce effects on performance are ingested.

Fluid balance and thermoregulation

About 75–80% of the chemical energy liberated during substrate oxidation appears as heat. In an activity such as running on the flat, the rate of heat production is a function of speed and the athlete's body mass. If the rate of heat production exceeds the rate of heat loss from the body, as is normally the case during running, body temperature will rise. The direction of heat exchange between the body and the environment depends on skin temperature and climatic conditions, but heat is gained by physical transfer in hot conditions. Evaporation of sweat is, then, the only available avenue of heat loss.

The rate of heat production during exercise is a function of the metabolic rate and declines as the race distance increases. In middle distance races the rate of heat production is high but the duration is short, so although there is a substantial increase in muscle temperature only small changes in core temperature occur. In longer races, however, hyperthermia and dehydration consequent upon sweat loss are potentially major problems to a runner, even to the extent of

fatality (see Chapter 6). Heat exhaustion and collapse occur most often on hot days, but even at moderate (23 °C) environmental temperatures, rectal temperature may be elevated above 40 °C in marathon runners. Many of the highest values of rectal temperature recorded in distance runners have been found after races at intermediate distances. Among competitors in a 14-km road race, Sutton (1990) reported more than 30 cases over a period of years where rectal temperature exceeded 42 °C. These data suggest that hyperthermia may be more common when the rate of heat production is very high (see Chapter 6). At very high exercise intensities skin blood flow is likely to be reduced, with a larger fraction of the cardiac output being directed to the working muscles, so heat loss will be reduced.

Severe hyperthermia is associated with a reduction in the ability to continue running. It has been proposed that exercise is terminated when a critical core temperature is reached. While this may be true for prolonged exercise in the heat, it does not appear to be true when the ambient temperature is low. It has been shown that there is an optimum temperature for the performance of prolonged exercise and that this is about 10 °C for exercise of about 60–90 min duration. The optimum temperature will, of course, depend on a number of factors other than the exercise duration: these factors include the rate of metabolic heat production, which is a function of running speed, the prevailing wind velocity, and the clothing worn as well as the anthropometric and physiological characteristics of the individual. Among runners it is well recognized that performance is impaired in conditions of high temperature and humidity; this recognition is usually translated into a more cautious pace, helping to reduce the incidence of heat illness.

The secondary problem of dehydration resulting from prolonged sweating may be a more significant issue. In conditions of high temperature and humidity, sweat losses are high even when the exercise duration is short. In the shorter middle distance events sweat loss is negligible, but performance is reduced by prior dehydration, and athletes competing in these events may be dehydrated prior to exercise if proper attention is not paid to replacement of losses. In more prolonged exercise sweat losses may be large, resulting in significant losses of body water and electrolytes, especially sodium (see Chapter 6). The rate of sweat loss during distance running is generally in excess of the rate at which fluid is consumed, so some degree of hypohydration normally occurs. Even in the same race and with the same fluid intake, however, there is a large variation between runners in the extent of sweat loss; this may vary from 1 to 6% of body mass in a marathon run in moderate environmental conditions. Dehydration results in a greater impairment of endurance events that rely primarily on aerobic metabolism than in those events where there is a significant contribution from anaerobic metabolism. This hypothesis is supported by the results of a study which showed that pre-exercise dehydration equal to about 2% of body mass resulted in a 3.1% reduction in performance in a 1500-m race compared with a 6.3% reduction in a 10-km race (Armstrong *et al.* 1985). The factors influencing fluid and electrolyte homeostasis during exercise and the effects of disturbances in fluid balance on exercise performance have been the subject of extensive reviews (see Maughan & Shirreffs 1998).

Nutritional limitations to performance

The role of diet in training and competition is covered in detail in Chapter 5 and will be discussed only briefly here. During periods of intensive training the energy demand will be high and food intake must be increased to meet this demand (Fig. 2.5).

The fuels used for energy production in distance running are fat and carbohydrate, with only a very small (about 5%) contribution from protein. There is an increased reliance on carbohydrate as a fuel as the intensity of effort increases, and the contribution of fat oxidation to energy metabolism in middle distance races is negligible. Because the demand for carbohydrate is high and the body's carbohydrate stores are limited, the diet must supply sufficient carbohydrate or performance will suffer. Many laboratory studies using bicycle exercise have shown a close association between the point at which the glycogen content of the exercising muscles falls close to zero and the subjective feeling of exhaustion. Studies using running exercise also show a fall in the muscle glycogen content, but significant amounts remain even at the point of exhaustion. For example, Sherman *et al.* (1981) measured the glycogen content of the gastrocnemius muscle after a 20.9-km time trial (mean

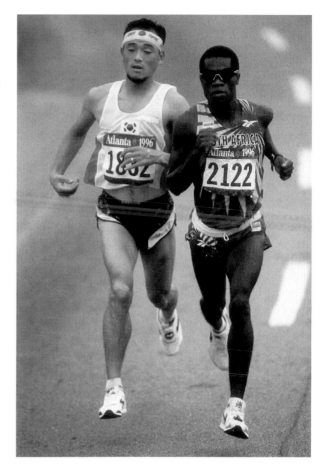

Fig. 2.5 Long distance runners are less muscular and consequently lighter than other track athletes. Their leg muscles possess a majority of type I (slow twitch) fibres. Such a profile may reflect the training patterns of these athletes. Lee Bong-Ju of Korea (left) silver medalist, and Josia Thugwane (South Africa) gold medal winner of the Olympic marathon, Atlanta, 1996. © Allsport / G.M. Prior.

running time 83 min) and found postexercise muscle glycogen values were only reduced by about 50–65% of the pre-exercise value. After a 30-km race, muscle glycogen content falls to about 30% of the pre-exercise value (Karlsson & Saltin 1971). However, when a high carbohydrate diet was fed in the few days prior to exercise the pre-exercise glycogen stores were increased by 100% and the postexercise glycogen content was actually greater than the pre-exercise value observed after the runners consumed their normal diet. These results suggest that muscle glycogen depletion may be a less likely candidate for

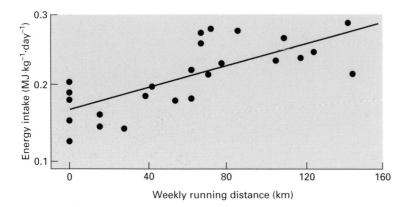

Fig. 2.6 Total energy intake increases with the volume of training carried out. A statistically significant relationship is observed between these two variables even without correction for body weight. Expression of energy intake relative to body weight increases the closeness of the relationship.

the limitation of exercise performance in running than in cycling. Again, however, the possibility of a limitation imposed by glycogen depletion in a specific fibre type cannot be ignored.

In middle distance running, the rate of glycogen breakdown is high, but the duration is short; although it might be possible to use more than 100 g of muscle glycogen during a race over a distance of 1609 m (1 mile), the total muscle glycogen content is likely to be at least 350 g, so glycogen availability should not be limiting. However, there is some evidence to suggest that performance in exercise of only a few minutes' duration is also influenced by the availability of carbohydrate as a metabolic fuel.

Although it is common for marathon runners to consume a high carbohydrate diet in the days prior to a race, there have been relatively few studies where the effects of carbohydrate feeding, either before or during exercise, have been investigated using running rather than cycling exercise. In the study referred to previously (Karlsson & Saltin 1971) it appeared that runners in a 30-km race slowed down less in the later stages of the race if they had consumed a high-carbohydrate diet in the days prior to the race; there was no difference between the trials in running speed at the beginning of the race, but the overall performance time was better after the high-carbohydrate diet. Ingestion of carbohydrate during treadmill running can extend the running time at a fixed speed and can allow runners to maintain a higher speed in the later stages of a long run. These results suggest that the availability of carbohydrate as a metabolic fuel may limit performance during prolonged running. Nutritional strategies to increase carbohydrate storage

and training strategies to spare carbohydrate use are described elsewhere in this book (see Chapter 5).

References

Armstrong, L.E., Costill, D.L. & Fink, W.J. (1985) Influence of diuretic-induced dehydration on competitive running performance. *Medicine and Science in Sports and Exercise* **17**, 456–461.

Costill, D.L., Bowers, R. & Kammer, W.F. (1970) Skinfold estimates of body fat among marathon runners. *Medicine and Science in Sports* **2**, 93–95.

Coyle, E.F., Hopper, M.K. & Coggan, A.R. (1990) Maximal oxygen uptake relative to plasma, expansion. *International Journal of Sports Medicine* **11**, 116–119.

Davies, C.T.M. & Thompson, M.W. (1979) Aerobic performance of female marathon and male ultramarathon athletes. *European Journal of Applied Physiology* **41**, 233–245.

Eichner, E.R. (1992) Sports anemia, iron supplements, and blood doping. *Medicine and Science in Sports and Exercise* **24**, S315–S318.

Henriksson, J. & Hickner, R.C. (1992) Skeletal muscle adaptations to endurance training. In: *Intermittent High Intensity Exercise* (ed. D.A.D. Macleod), pp. 5–25. Spon, London.

Housh, T.J., Thorland, W.G., Johnson, G.O., Hughes, R.A. & Cisra, C.J. (1986) Body composition and body build variables as predictors of middle distance running performance. *Journal of Sports Medicine* **26**, 258–262.

Karlsson, J. & Saltin, B. (1971) Diet, muscle glycogen and endurance performance. *Journal of Applied Physiology* **31**, 203–206.

Martin, D.E., May, D.F. & Pilbeam, S.P. (1985) Ventilation limitations to performance among elite male distance runners. In: *The 1984 Olympic Scientific Congress Proceedings*, Vol. 3 (ed. D.M. Landers), pp. 121–131. Human Kinetics Publishers, Champaign.

Maughan, R.J. (1990) Marathon running. In: *Physiology of Sports* (ed. T. Reilly), pp. 121–152. Spon, London.

Maughan, R.J. (1992) Aerobic function. In: *Sport Science Review* (ed. R.J. Shephard), pp. 28–42. Human Kinetics, Champaign.

Maughan, R.J. (1994) Physiology and nutrition for middle distance and long distance running. In: *Perspectives in Exercise Science and Sports Medicine*, Vol. 7. *Physiology and Nutrition in Competitive Sport* (eds D.R. Lamb, H.J. Knuttgen & R. Murray), pp. 329–371. Cooper, Carmel, Indiana.

Maughan, R.J. & Greenhaff, P.L. (1991) High intensity exercise and acid–base balance: the influence of diet and induced metabolic alkalosis on performance. In: *Advances in Nutrition and Top Sport* (ed. F. Brouns), pp. 145–165. Karger, Basel.

Maughan, R.J. & Leiper, J.B. (1983) Aerobic capacity and fractional utilization of aerobic capacity in elite and nonelite male and female marathon runners. *European Journal of Applied Physiology* **52**, 80–87.

Maughan, R.J. & Shirreffs, S.M. (1998) Fluid and electrolyte loss and replacement in exercise. In: *Oxford Textbook of Sports Medicine* (eds M. Harries, C. Williams, W.D. Stanish & L.L. Micheli), 2nd edn, pp. 97–113. Oxford University Press, New York.

Medbo, J.I., Mohn, A.C., Tabata, I. *et al.* (1988) Anaerobic capacity determined by maximal accumulated O_2 deficit. *Journal of Applied Physiology* **64**, 50–60.

Pate, R.R., Sparling, P.B., Wilson, G.E., Cureton, K.J. & Miller, B.J. (1987) Cardiorespiratory and metabolic responses to submaximal and maximal exercise in elite women distance runners. *International Journal of Sports Medicine* **8**, 91–95S.

Peronnet, F. & Thibault, G. (1989) Mathematical analysis of running performance and world records. *Journal of Applied Physiology* **67**, 453–465.

Saltin, B., Henriksson, J., Nygaard, E., Andersen, P. & Jansson, E. (1977) Fibre types and metabolic potentials of skeletal muscles in sedentary man and endurance runners. *Annals of the New York Academy of Sciences* **301**, 3–29.

Scott, B.K. & Houmard, J.A. (1994) Peak running velocity is highly related to distance running performance. *International Journal of Sports Medicine* **15**, 504–507.

Sherman, W.M., Costill, D.L., Fink, W.J. & Miller, J.M. (1981) Effect of exercise–diet manipulation on muscle glycogen and its subsequent utilisation during performance. *International Journal of Sports Medicine* **2**, 114–118.

Sjodin, B. & Svedenhag, J. (1985) Applied physiology of marathon running. *Sports Medicine* **2**, 83–99.

Snell, P. (1990) Middle distance running. In: *Physiology of Sports* (ed. T. Reilly), pp. 101–120. Spon, London.

Sutton, J.R. (1990) Clinical implications of fluid imbalance. In *Perspectives in Exercise Science and Sports Medicine*, Vol. 3. *Fluid Homeostasis During Exercise* (eds C.V. Gisolfi & D.R. Lamb), pp. 425–448. Benchmark, Carmel, Indiana.

Recommended reading

Maughan, R.J. (1994) Physiology and nutrition for middle distance and long distance running. In: *Perspectives in Exercise Science and Sports Medicine,* Vol. 7. *Physiology and Nutrition in Competitive Sport* (eds D.R. Lamb, H.J. Knuttgen & R. Murray), pp. 329–371. Cooper, Carmel, Indiana.

Sjodin, B. & Svedenhag, J. (1985) Applied physiology of marathon running. *Sports Medicine* **2**, 83–99.

Snell, P. (1990) Middle distance running. In: *Physiology of Sports* (ed. T. Reilly), pp. 101–120. Spon, London.

Chapter 3

Biomechanics of running

The study of the forces that act on the body and the body movements during running provide an insight into how certain changes in running technique influence running performance, and how a number of biomechanical parameters can predispose a runner to injury. This chapter will describe the biomechanics of running, focusing on the movement of the lower limb segments and the forces encountered during each foot strike with the ground. The effect of running speed and running surface on specific biomechanical parameters and their subsequent influence on running injuries will be reviewed, and the implications of these findings for the design of appropriate footwear discussed.

Kinematics of running

Sagittal plane kinematics of the lower extremity

Lower extremity sagittal plane kinematics during running involve flexion and extension of the hip, knee, ankle and metatarsophalangeal joints. In 1975 Dillman reviewed sagittal plane kinematics during running as a function of running speed, focusing primarily on the relationships between stride length and stride rate, and displacements of the centre of gravity. A decade later Williams (1985) presented an extensive review of lower extremity kinematics during running and, in particular, documented the effects of running speed on kinematics. The reader is referred to these excellent reviews for a comprehensive discussion of their work. In this section, the sagittal plane kinematics presented by these workers is summarized for the support phase of running.

Hip joint

At foot strike the hip is flexed between 25 and 30° and changes little during the time immediately after ground contact. Figure 3.1a shows that the thigh of the subject is in 26° of flexion at heel strike. The thigh remains in that position for at least 65 ms before beginning to extend. Midway through the support phase of the stride, the hip begins extending along with the knee and ankle joint. The thigh is in 22° of extension at toe off (Fig. 3.1a). Extension of these joints then continues through to toe off, at which point the hip is in about 20° of extension. At faster running speeds, when greater propulsive forces are developed, hip extension at take off may increase by a further 5°.

Knee joint

The knee is not fully extended at foot strike, being flexed by more than 10°. A further 20–30° of flexion occurs early in the support period as the vertical velocity of the runner's foot is reduced and the force of ground impact is cushioned.

As the hip, knee and ankle joints begin to extend during the latter half of the support period, the foot pushes against the running surface and the body's centre of gravity accelerates upward and forward. The knee does not go into full extension during the latter part of the support phase but remains in 15–20° of flexion (Fig. 3.1a).

Knee flexion during the early part of the support phase of running is a natural mechanism that cushions some of the force of impact. Although the peak impact forces with the ground increase with increasing running velocity (discussed below), a clear relationship between knee joint flexion and running velocity has yet to be established. Indeed, maximum knee flexion during the support phase may only increase a few degrees with increased running speed.

Ankle joint

Different foot strike patterns can greatly influence ankle movement patterns and both dorsiflexed and plantarflexed ankles have been observed at foot strike. Most runners initially contact the running surface with their rearfoot and, for these runners, initial

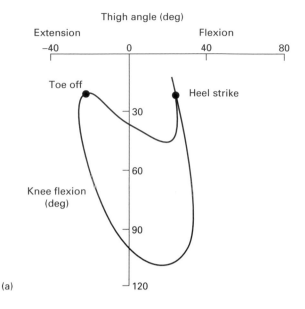

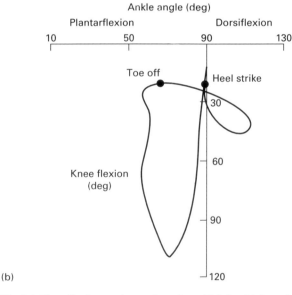

Fig. 3.1 Knee flexion angle as a function of (a) the thigh angle and (b) the ankle angle for a complete stride of running at a speed of 3.8 m·s⁻¹. Thigh angle is expressed relative to vertical. Data from Milliron and Cavanagh (1990).

contact is made with their ankle plantarflexed approximately 5°. Figure 3.1b demonstrates the relationship between ankle and knee motion during weight bearing. Immediately after heel strike there is another few

degrees of plantarflexion, followed by 15–20° of dorsiflexion. In the latter half of the support phase, as the knee extends, the ankle plantarflexes up to 30° before toe off.

Investigation of plantar flexor muscle length characteristics and muscle activity characteristics have shown that the plantar flexor muscles of the calf primarily act eccentrically to control ankle dorsiflexion during support (Milliron & Cavanagh 1990). Concentric activity occurs only in the first 15–20% of the support period. Given that the primary mechanism for tendinitis injuries is eccentric overload (see Chapter 0), it is likely that there might be a strong relationship between the incidence of Achilles tendinitis in runners and the amount of eccentric activity of the plantar flexors.

This hypothesis has important practical implications for the role of footwear in injury reduction, because ankle joint motion and Achilles tendon elongation can be influenced by the design of the running shoe midsole. For example, increasing the thickness of a running shoe midsole under the heel reduces the amount of dorsiflexion at a time when the Achilles tendon is strained under eccentric muscle loads. Alternatively, making the rear of a running shoe stiffer will reduce the compression of the midsole during weight bearing, and similarly reduce dorsiflexion at a time when the Achilles tendon is under eccentric loading. Designing the midsole under the heel to be both stiffer and thicker will reduce dorsiflexion which, in turn, will reduce the potential loads on the Achilles tendon without sacrificing shoe cushioning.

Metatarsophalangeal joint

During barefoot running the metatarsophalangeal joints dorsiflex about 30° during the last half of the support phase. However, when running in shoes the range of motion of the metatarsophalangeal joints will be greatly influenced by the shoe design. Running shoes are designed with toe spring in order to facilitate toe off. Toe spring refers to the gradual increase in the elevation of the sole of the shoe off a flat surface from the ball region to the tip of the shoe (Fig. 3.2). Using running shoes with toe spring causes a slight dorsiflexion of the metatarsophalangeal joints, resulting in reduced dorsiflexion of the metatarsophalangeal joints during the push-off phase. Increasing

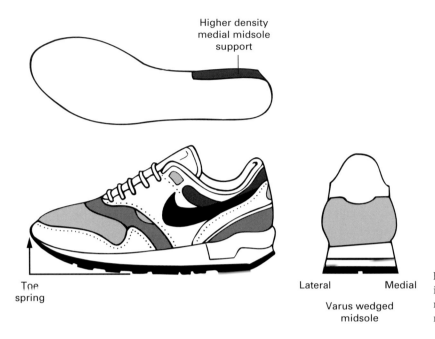

Higher density medial midsole support

Toe spring

Lateral   Medial

Varus wedged midsole

Fig. 3.2 Running shoe design showing toe spring, higher density medial midsole support and a varus wedged midsole.

the flexibility of a running shoe at the point where the metatarsophalangeal joints flex will also influence the amount of joint dorsiflexion during the latter stance phase. This flexibility is usually achieved by moulding grooves into the outsole pattern of a shoe and/or into the midsole along a line aligned with the metatarsophalangeal joints.

Frontal plane kinematics of the rearfoot

Running is often considered to be a straight-line activity, with movement of the limb segments occurring only in the plane of progression (the sagittal plane). However, lower extremity movements that occur at right angles to this plane (the frontal plane) should also be considered. In fact, movement of the rearfoot relative to the shank or the forefoot has a greater influence on many running injuries and the design of running footwear than sagittal plane limb motions.

Increases in walking speed are attained by increasing both stride rate and stride length. However, increasing stride rate is the most important contributor to increasing velocity. For example, a 1 m·s⁻¹ increase in walking speed—from 1.5 m·s⁻¹ to 2.5 m·s⁻¹—is achieved by a 44% increase in stride rate and a 15% increase in stride length (Fig. 3.3). At a speed of *c.* 2.3 m·s⁻¹, the transition from walking to running

occurs because it becomes more economical to run rather than walk (Alexander 1992). Once running, further increases in running speed are achieved primarily by increasing stride length (see Fig. 3.3).

At the long stride lengths attained when running —which can be twice as long as walking strides— rotation of the ball and socket type hip joint aligns the leg with the midline of the body at foot strike. As there is no force on the foot during the swing phase, the pronounced hip rotation causes the rearfoot to be in a supinated orientation at foot strike. This causes the foot and shoe to make first contact with the ground along the outside edge. Immediately following foot strike there is a rapid pronation of the foot at the subtalar joint as impact force develops. It is commonly believed that excessive pronation is a risk factor associated with many of the more prevalent overuse running injuries, including runner's knee, Achilles tendinitis, anterior tibial stress syndrome and plantar fasciitis.

Two-dimensional rearfoot eversion

Although pronation at the subtalar joint involves motion in the frontal and horizontal planes and is associated with ankle dorsiflexion (three-dimensional motion), two-dimensional analysis of rearfoot

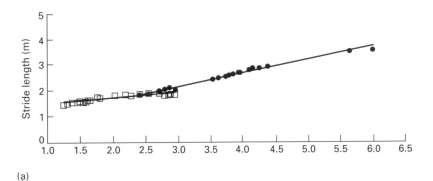

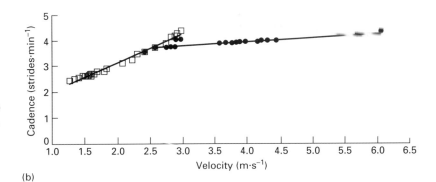

Fig. 3.3 (a) Stride length and (b) stride rate at walking speeds (□) and distance running speeds (●) for a single subject. The lines represent lines of best fit (linear regressions). A stride is defined to be a complete cycle involving a step by both right and left legs.

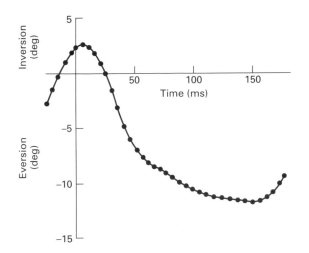

Fig. 3.4 Orientation of the rearfoot in a frontal plane relative to the long axis of the shank during the support phase of running. The angle is referenced to the orientation of the two segments during standing. Heel strike occurs at time 0.

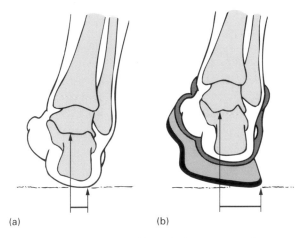

Fig. 3.5 The moment arm of frontal plane eversion for running (a) barefoot and (b) in shoes with cushioned midsoles.

eversion relative to the shank (in the frontal plane) can provide valuable insight into the biomechanics of running. Figure 3.4 shows how the rearfoot moves from inversion through to greater amounts of eversion during the support phase of running. If the axis of rearfoot eversion coincides with the midline of the calcaneus and talus (Fig. 3.5a), the initial point of contact between the heel and running surface creates a turning moment, which tends to evert the rearfoot. For an athlete running in shoes the thickness of the midsole material beneath the rearfoot increases the length of the moment arm upon which the impact force acts on the inversion–eversion axis (Fig. 3.5a). This explains why running in shoes usually results in more pronation than running barefoot.

Manipulating the length of the moment arm by designing a flare on the medial and lateral edges of the midsole (Fig. 3.5b) can influence the amount of rearfoot eversion. A 15° flare on the lateral side of the midsole increases the width at the bottom of a 24-mm thick midsole in the rearfoot by 6 mm. Increasing the width in this area where the initial contact with the running surface is made increases the eversion moment arm. However, an equivalent flare on the medial side of the rearfoot midsole increases the inversion moment opposing rearfoot eversion once the pronating foot develops pressure beneath the medial aspect of the heel. A negative flare on the lateral side reduces the eversion moment arm. Indeed, research has shown that a midsole flared on both medial and lateral sides reduces rearfoot eversion (Clarke et al. 1983). On the other hand, Nigg and Morlock (1987) found that a running shoe flared 16° on just the lateral side did not result in a decreased amount of rearfoot eversion, nor a decreased maximum rate of eversion during the support phase of running at a speed of 4 m·s⁻¹. They did demonstrate, however, that rounding the lateral edge of the rear midsole to create the equivalent of a negative heel flare and a narrower width resulted in decreased eversion and rate of eversion relative to a midsole with a vertical non-flared lateral edge (Nigg & Morlock 1987).

In the design of today's running shoes the feature most commonly incorporated to control eversion of the rearfoot is a section of firmer cushioning material in the medial half of the rear midsole. The firmer material may be confined to the side wall of the midsole, or it may extend a few millimetres beneath the medial heel region. The medial support may also be incorporated as a wedge (see Fig. 3.2). Wedging the midsole in a frontal cross-section with a uniform density of material significantly influences eversion of the rearfoot. Varus wedged midsoles from 8 to 10° can reduce maximum rearfoot eversion by up to 67% compared to identically constructed non-wedged shoes.

Dual density midsole designs and midsoles wedged in varus are adopted from the orthotics industry. Foot orthoses provide many different types of corrections to foot and leg function to compensate for anatomical or biomechanical anomalies. Using orthotics to change inversion–eversion angles of the rearfoot can be effective to relieve the low-grade pain associated with some running injuries (see Chapter 6). Consequently, the design of the modern running shoe attempts to control subtalar joint pronation in an effort to reduce the incidence of chronic running injuries. The effectiveness of orthotics for the control of excessive pronation and the alleviation of pain is a widely held clinical belief and, although not unequivocal, biomechanical research on the influence of in-shoe orthotics on running kinematics support their use to control rearfoot eversion when running.

Three-dimensional subtalar joint pronation

The axis of subtalar joint pronation is not in any of the conventional anatomical planes. Subtalar joint pronation is a three-dimensional motion involving rearfoot eversion in the frontal plane and external rotation relative to the tibia in the horizontal plane. These movements are associated with ankle joint dorsiflexion in the sagittal plane. It is generally accepted that measuring lower extremity kinematics three-dimensionally provides a more accurate description in addition to providing two other components of motion.

Three-dimensional analysis has characterized subtalar joint pronation during running in the following way (Engsberg & Andrews 1987). The first 10–11% of support is defined by plantar flexion of the combined talocalcaneal–talocrural joint eversion and minimal internal tibial rotation. In the next 37% of support eversion of combined talocalcaneal–talocrural joint dominates, accompanied by internal tibial rotation. Most, but not all, runners display eversion through the last half of the support period, somewhat contradicting conventional thinking that supination, or at least inversion, occurs in the later stage of stance. Comparison between three-dimensional and two-dimensional measurements show differences of up to 20% for the inversion–eversion component. Such differences are largely dependent upon running style as well as components of motion about other axes.

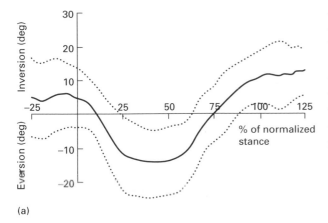

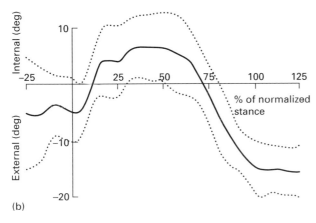

Fig. 3.6 Mean motion (solid lines) plus or minus one standard deviation (dotted lines) of the rearfoot relative to the shank in (a) the frontal plane and mean motion of the shank relative to the rearfoot in (b) the horizontal plane during the stance phase of running in shoes with a varus wedge insert to regulate pronation. Data from the Nike Sport Research Lab.

Rotations of the femur and the tibia around their long axes

The structure of the subtalar joint between the tibia and talus is such that any rearfoot eversion that occurs during pronation is accompanied by internal rotation of the tibia (Fig. 3.6). There is also external rotation of the femur because of external hip rotation during the stance phase of running. Because rotation of these long bones act in opposite directions, the potential exists for twisting torques to be generated at the knee joint which may expose the soft-tissue structures of

the knee joint to injury (Nigg & Cole 1994). However, there is a highly individual response to the susceptibility of knee injury from this mechanism. Individual differences in the position of the ankle and the loading of the foot during foot–ground contact, as well as the integrity of the ligaments of the ankle, determine the amount of internal rotation of the tibia. Nevertheless, the combination of excessive eversion of the rearfoot and the transfer of movement to internal rotation of the tibia is a predictor of overuse knee injury (Hintermann & Nigg 1998).

Kinetics of running

Measurement of the forces (kinetics) which underlie the movements of the body during running provide a direct indication of the loads to which the body is subjected at each foot–ground contact. Ground reaction force (GRF) characteristics, the pressure distribution on the plantar surface of the foot and the acceleration profiles of lower limb segments are commonly used in sport biomechanics to measure these loads. Each of these parameters is closely related. Foot contact generates a reaction force from the ground that is applied to the foot. This reaction force is distributed under the plantar surface of the foot and its effect is to accelerate individual body segments and transmit force to adjacent segments.

Ground reaction force

The force generated between the foot and the ground is commonly divided into three components acting at right angles (Fig. 3.7). The vertical component of GRF (F_z) opposes the downward motion of the body caused by gravity before propelling it upward for the next flight phase. The anteroposterior (AP) component of GRF acts in the direction of progression: it can either reduce or increase running velocity. The mediolateral (ML) component of GRF acts at a right angle to the direction of progression, thus being responsible for directional changes. The vertical component is by far the largest component followed, in order, by the AP and ML components (Fig. 3.8). In recreational athletes running at *c.* 3.75 m·s⁻¹, F_z, AP and ML peaks reach approximately 2.2, 0.5 and 0.2 of body weight (BW), respectively.

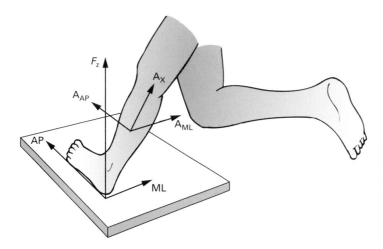

Fig. 3.7 The components of ground reaction force acting on the foot and components of segmental acceleration experienced by the shank during running. A_{AP}, anterioposterior acceleration; A_{ML}, mediolateral acceleration; A_X, axial acceleration; AP, anteroposterior force; F_z, vertical force; ML, mediolateral force.

Vertical component of GRF

F_z can be divided into impact (or passive) and propulsive (or active) components. The passive component of F_z describes the initial collision of the lower limb with the ground. It occurs within the first 50 ms of ground contact and is characterized by rapid rise and decay times (see Fig. 3.8). The active component represents the effort of the muscular system in controlling the vertical displacement of the body: it lasts the entire duration of foot–ground contact and displays a substantially slower rise and decay time but generally larger peak magnitudes than the passive component. It should be noted that the passive component of F_z does not imply an absence of muscular activity. Rather, it reflects the fact that the muscular activity that is initiated before ground contact cannot be modified in response to the rapid loading of impact. Of the two components of F_z the passive component is most often associated with injury. The active component of F_z has more commonly been examined from a performance perspective.

Runners who experience greater passive F_z peaks are more likely to get injured than those who experienced lower passive peaks (Nigg *et al.* 1984). Information obtained from research performed on animal models suggests that the *rate* of loading is even more important than force magnitude in the initiation of joint deterioration and progression to osteoarthritis. Consequently, for any given runner, higher passive F_z peaks and/or rates of loading are likely to increase the risk of injury.

The active component of F_z represents the upward thrust of the body by the locomotor system and the impulse associated with these forces cause changes in the body's vertical velocity. As running speed increases, larger changes in vertical velocity occur and runners trying to increase running speed may consequently increase the active component of F_z. Care should be taken not to produce disproportionately large vertical movement of the body because runners who show larger vertical oscillations at a given running speed have a higher energy cost than their counterparts with small movements of their centre of mass (Williams & Cavanagh 1987).

Horizontal component of GRF in anteroposterior direction

The AP component of GRF during running can be divided into braking and propulsion phases (see Fig. 3.8). Following touchdown and for half the duration of the ground contact, the AP force opposes the forward motion of the runner (i.e. braking). The AP force changes direction midway through the contact to become propulsive in nature (propulsion). The changes in velocity caused by braking and propulsion should be almost identical in submaximal steady-state running except for the slightly larger propulsion needed to overcome air resistance. The braking part of the horizontal GRF causes a 5% reduction in speed which must be compensated by the propulsive part to maintain running speed (Cavanagh & Lafortune 1980). As both braking and propulsive phases are

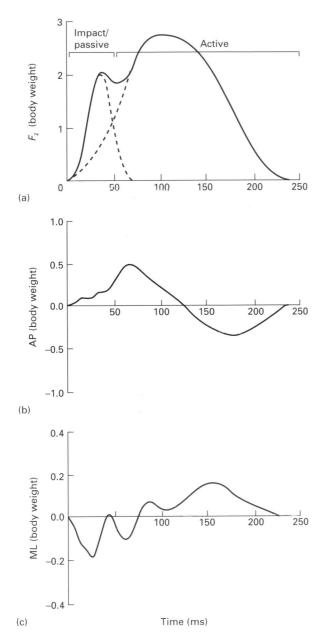

(a)

(b)

(c)   Time (ms)

Fig. 3.8 The typical force–time curves during running.
(a) Vertical force (F_z), (b) anteroposterior force (AP) and (c)
mediolateral force (ML). The passive or impact component of
F_z occurs during the first 50 ms and the active component
lasts for the entire foot–ground contact.

under muscular control, running techniques that
reduce braking should improve running efficiency.
Unfortunately, this rationale has not been supported
by biomechanical research (Williams & Cavanagh
1987), although data collected on a small number of
elite runners at velocities close to race pace reveal less
slowing down following foot–ground contact.

*Horizontal component of GRF in
mediolateral direction*

The component of GRF that is responsible for direction change (ML component) shows considerable
variability between runners. Even in straight-line running where the summation of consecutive ML velocity
changes must add up to zero, there is considerable
variability in the size of the force peaks, the number
of times the force changes direction and the impulse
causing directional change. In some runners small
non-zero resultant impulse from individual steps
occur, indicating zigzagging about the line of progression, thus suggesting inefficient running technique.
However, the link between running efficiency and
ML force has yet to be established experimentally.

Centre of pressure of GRF

The centre of pressure (CoP) represents the point of
application of the resultant GRF acting on the foot. As
such, it provides information about the structures of
the foot that are loaded during foot–ground contact.
Runners are classified into two groups based upon
the location of the initial contact of their foot/shoe
with the ground (Fig. 3.9). Approximately 70% of runners make ground contact with the posterior third of
their foot (rearfoot strikers) while the remaining 30%
make the initial contact with the middle third of their
foot (midfoot strikers). Centre of pressure analysis
indicates that the loading of the foot migrates progressively from the heel to the forefoot in rearfoot strikers.
In forefoot strikers, the CoP analysis shows that the
loading moves initially toward the heel before turning
and moving toward the ball of the foot.

Grouping of runners according to foot strike type
has shown specific GRF characteristics associated
with each foot strike type. Compared to rearfoot
strikers, GRF patterns of midfoot strikers show
smaller passive F_z peaks associated with impact.

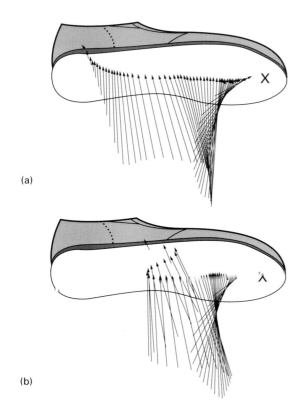

(a)

(b)

Fig. 3.9 The force vectors acting under the foot during running. (a) Pattern for rearfoot strikers: the initial contact occurs in the posterior third of the shoe. (b) Pattern for midfoot strikers: the initial contact occurs in the middle third of the shoe. Adapted from Cavanagh and Lafortune (1980).

Biomechanical research has not been able to demonstrate any consistent difference in the AP braking force characteristics of rearfoot and forefoot strikers. The F_z rate of loading and change in running velocity caused by initial braking impulse do not differ between rearfoot and midfoot strikers despite the differences in weight-bearing structures and loading patterns at foot strike.

Effects of running velocity

As running velocity increases, the impact peak and the rate of loading of the vertical GRF increases. The impact peak increases almost linearly for running velocities between 3 and 6 $m \cdot s^{-1}$; at sprinting speed impact peaks as high as 5.2 BW have been recorded.

Although biomechanical researchers have used many different techniques to determine the rate of loading of F_z, all methods show that the rate of loading increases exponentially with increases in running velocity. Thus, faster running velocities are exposing the musculoskeletal system to greater risk of injury. More specifically, midtarsal and metatarsal structures are at greater risk because the CoP indicates that F_z impact peaks move anteriorly with increasing running velocity. These risks are further compounded by the fact that these structures are also responsible for transmitting the active component of F_z to the ground. The latter can reach 3.25 BW and 5.2 BW running at 6 $m \cdot s^{-1}$ and sprinting, respectively.

Effects of running surfaces

Runners adapt their running mechanics to the surface upon which they are running. Because of the technical constraints of force platform mounting, few researchers have examined the effects of different surfaces (grass, sand, asphalt) and slopes (different levels of incline and decline) on GRF variables. However, insight into some of the effects of surface types on GRF variables have been made by laying grass, asphalt and concrete on a Kistler force platform (Feehery 1986). It was found that there were lower passive and active F_z peaks on concrete than either on grass or asphalt, with no differences between the last two surfaces. These results are unexpected and, although difficulties in data collection caution care when interpreting the results, similar investigations measuring lower limb acceleration support the notion that running on grass causes greater loads than running on concrete.

Investigation of the effect of surface stiffness on F_z by using tracks with different numbers of rubber layers has shown that surface stiffness has no effect on the active component of F_z. This has been attributed to the ability of the runners to adapt their leg stiffness to offset the changes in surface stiffness and it has been suggested that it may underlie the hypothesized enhanced performance of middle- and long-distance runners on compliant running tracks.

Downhill running exposes runners to substantially higher F_z impact peaks than level running, and the AP component associated with braking also changes dramatically. For example, running down an 8.3% gradient increases the F_z impact peak by 14% while the braking impulse is almost double the propulsive impulse. The point of impact between the ground and the foot also moves further towards the back of the foot.

Effects of footwear

From an injury prevention perspective, the role of the midsole in running footwear is to reduce GRF peaks and force rates of loading. This can be accomplished without adversely affecting the heel region of the shoe. The use of softer and/or thicker materials should lead to lower passive peaks and rates of loading. Care should be taken when using softer midsoles as 'bottoming out' could lead to the opposite effect, higher force peaks and rates of loading.

The protection of the forefoot region is more problematic as any reduction in force translates into a reduction in propulsive thrust. Thus, the use of softer and/or thicker midsoles to reduce loading could lead to sluggish propulsion. Furthermore, thicker midsoles reduce forefoot flexibility, which would require runners to waste valuable energy bending their shoes. It has also been suggested that reduced forefoot flexibility increases the risk of injuries such as plantar fasciitis. The pressure distribution maps presented in the next section will be used to suggest a solution that offers protection without impeding performance.

Numerous biomechanical investigations have attempted to measure the cushioning effects of footwear midsole properties on F_z. The consensus is that midsole properties have minimal effects on F_z. This near absence of effect may also be explained by the runners' ability to adjust their leg stiffness to maintain preferred running mechanics. It should be noted, however, that running in footwear results in a substantial reduction in F_z peak and rate of loading compared to barefoot running.

Plantar pressure

Measurement of plantar pressure

Plantar pressure profiles offer a visual description of how force is distributed under the foot, as well as providing quantitative information about the timing and loading magnitude of individual foot structures. Plantar pressure can be recorded either with insoles that contain arrays of sensors that measure the entire plantar surface of the foot, or with individual discrete sensors which can be mounted at specified locations of interest. Both technologies measure the loading that is applied perpendicular to the plantar surface of the foot. The feet change orientation with respect to the ground during the stance phase of running, from a toes up position at foot–ground contact, to heel up position at toe off. Thus, the loading measured with the pressure sensors does not correspond to the vertical component of GRF measured with force platforms.

Plantar pressure profiles

During barefoot running at speeds of c. 4 m·s^{-1} (Fig. 3.10), when the foot contacts the ground the pressure under the heel peaks in c. 15 ms.

Some 15 ms later, pressure under the forefoot and the toes can be detected. The pressure under the metatarsal heads exceeds the pressure under the heel from 60 ms until toe off. Peak forefoot pressures are not reached until 120–140 ms which coincides almost exactly with the time the heel lifts off the ground. Compared to the information gathered from the centre of pressure paths measured with force platform, the pressure maps indicate a definite propulsive involvement of the big toe (hallux) during the later phase of foot–ground contact.

Pressure-measuring insoles produce in excess of 2500 distinct data points during a single running step. To convey this information in a condensed format, maps of peak pressure are commonly used by biomechanists. They show the distribution of the pressure peaks under the foot having areas of high pressure located in the heel and forefoot areas (see Fig. 3.10). At a running speed of 4 m·s^{-1} the peak pressure under the metatarsal heads is slightly higher than the pressure under the heel (330–335 kPa vs. 312 kPa). A close examination of the peak map reveals a crease between the metatarsal heads and the toes. The pressure peaks are more or less equal under the hallux and the metatarsal heads but lower under the other toes.

Some researchers have used discrete sensors to estimate the relative load-bearing and propulsion functions of different foot structures during shod treadmill running (Hennig *et al.* 1996). The results of such analysis reveal that the first metatarsal head (21%) followed by the hallux (17%) and the third

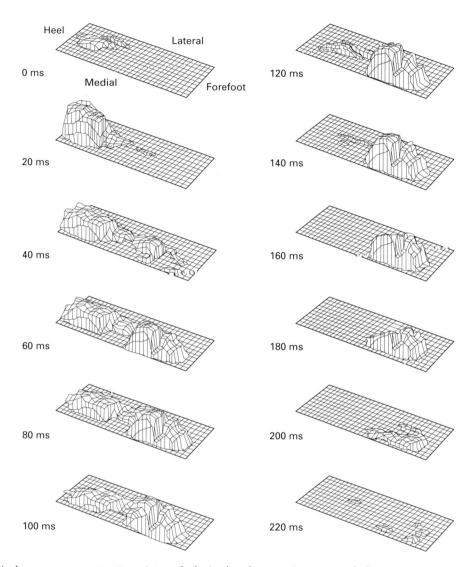

Fig. 3.10 Typical pressure maps at *c.* 15 ms intervals during barefoot running at a speed of 4 m·s⁻¹.

metatarsal head (14.6%) played major load-bearing functions during running. The other five structures (lateral and medial heel, lateral and medial midfoot, and fifth metatarsal head) each contributed between 7 and 11% to load bearing.

Effects of running velocity

Plantar pressure measurements have also been used to examine the effects of running velocity on foot loading. As running velocity increases the peak plantar

pressures also increase. The largest increases in peak pressure occur under the lateral and central part of the heel and under the hallux. These findings further support the observations of coaches that increases in running velocity are usually associated with an increased risk of injury.

Effects of footwear

Footwear plays an important part in reducing the pressure under the foot during running (Fig. 3.11).

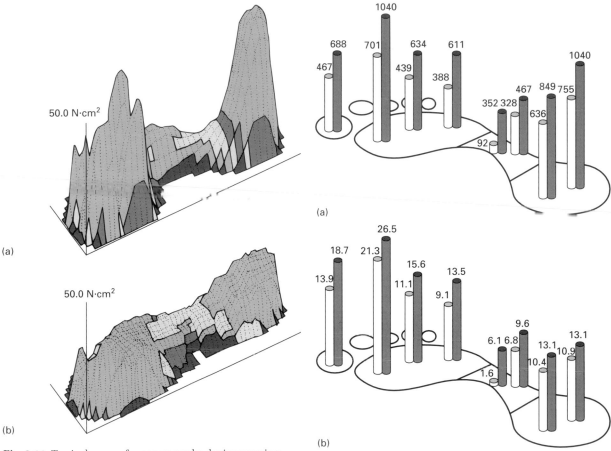

Fig. 3.11 Typical maps of pressure peaks during running. (a) Barefoot running and (b) shod running.

Fig. 3.12 (a) The ranges of pressure peaks (in kPa) recorded under eight anatomical structures with 19 different running shoe models and (b) the range of relative loads applied to these structures (%). Adapted from Hennig and Milani (1995).

The pressure peaks under the heel, metatarsal heads and hallux during barefoot running (Fig. 3.11a) are reduced by almost 50% when running in shoes (Fig. 3.11b), largely by spreading the loading over a greater area. For instance, the deformation of the shoe midsole allows the metatarsal heads to act more like a unit than five individual structures. Also the loading area under the midfoot is widened and the arch contributes to the weight-bearing function of the foot when shoes are worn.

Footwear construction can also alter pressure profiles and the relative loading of different foot structures. Measuring peak pressure under the head of the first metatarsal in 19 different shoe models, Hennig and Milani (1995) found differences in pressure of up to 340 kPa (Fig. 3.12). Direct comparison of footwear using relative loading revealed that different

constructions can significantly modify how the foot functions. As illustrated in Fig. 3.13, shoe A caused a greater involvement of the hallux and first metatarsal in propulsion, while shoe B caused a shift of the propulsion toward the third and fifth metatarsal bones.

The concentration of high pressure under the metatarsal heads confirms the need for protection of these structures by footwear. As previously discussed, this need for protection must be addressed without sacrificing performance which is characterized by the propulsive force: rather than reducing the overall pressure or GRF, footwear must prevent localized pressure points by distributing plantar loading across

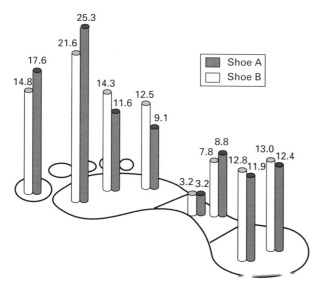

Fig. 3.13 The mean relative load patterns produced by two different running shoe models. Adapted from Hennig and Milani (1995).

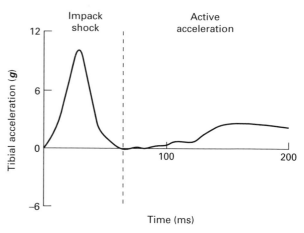

Fig. 3.14 The tibial axial acceleration during ground contact phase of running. Adapted from Lafortune and Hennig (1991).

the forefoot. Pressure maps recorded running barefoot and in different shoes reveal that shoes are successful in reducing the pressure under the metatarsal heads, although there are large differences between makes of shoe in this regard. Pressure maps have also shown that different shoe models can alter foot mechanics, which may lead to either the relief of pain, the onset of pain or overuse injuries. Consequently, runners must exercise great care in choosing footwear that address their individual performance and protection needs.

Pressure maps indicate a high involvement of the hallux during the later stage of foot–ground contact. Considering the position of the foot during this period, the involvement of the hallux implies the production of both vertical and shear propulsive force components. Thus, from a performance perspective it supports the importance of providing the corresponding area of the shoe outer sole with traction elements. This may be even more critical for racing footwear, as faster running velocities increase the propulsive role of the hallux and other toes.

Segmental acceleration and shock transmission

Segment acceleration, like GRF, can be divided into three components acting at right angles: axial (AX),

mediolateral (ML) and anteroposterior (AP) (see Fig. 3.7). Unlike the GRF components, the acceleration components change their orientation as the segment rotates in space; therefore AX, ML and AP accelerations do not coincide exactly with F_z, AP and ML forces during the stance phase of running. Most biomechanical research undertaken on segmental acceleration characteristics during running is on the axial component of tibial acceleration, and hence is the focus of this section.

Measurement of acceleration

While methodological difficulties of acceleration measurement make it difficult to compare directly across the many biomechanical studies in the area, common trends have emerged from these investigations. The axial signal measured by an accelerometer attached to the tibia can be ascribed to three sources: gravity (Ag), rotation (Ar) and impact ground reaction force (Ai). The passive and active features of the vertical GRF are reflected in the tibial axial acceleration characteristics. The passive GRF component causes the different segments of a runner's body to experience a transient shock. This shock occurs within the initial 30–50 ms of foot–ground contact and it features a sharp peak in acceleration with rapid rise and decay (Fig. 3.14). The active GRF component is responsible for the second less distinctive peak occurring later during ground contact. At the tibia, the shock peak can be as much as three times higher than the second active peak (Lafortune & Hennig 1991).

Although it is difficult to interpret individual axial acceleration measurements in terms of improved performance or risk of injury, it is commonly accepted that the shock component of acceleration can lead to musculoskeletal injuries. Indeed, the propagation of shock through the body may be a significant factor in the development of degenerative changes in joint and articular cartilage (Voloshin 1988).

Shock transmission

The shock originates in the foot before being transmitted to the lower leg, the thigh and the trunk, reaching the head 6–8 ms later (Valiant 1990). As it travels from segment to segment the magnitude of the shock is reduced (Lafortune *et al.* 1996). Tibial axial acceleration commonly reaches between 7 and 11.5 g when running at 3.8 m·s^{-1} (Clarke *et al.* 1985; Perry & Lafortune 1995). The variability in peak acceleration at this speed is attributed to differences in running mechanics, running surfaces and footwear.

Researchers have shown that runners who change their stride length either 10% above or below their preferred (optimal) stride length can experience similar variations in tibial axial shocks. (Hamill *et al.* 1994). These results suggest that running with shorter strides can reduce the risk of lower limb injuries but impose greater disturbance to the visual and vestibular functions.

Effects of running velocity and running surface

Similar to its effect on GRF characteristics, running velocity has been shown to markedly affect tibial shock. Higher running velocities result in greater tibial shock. For example, an increase in running speed from 3.35 to 5.26 m·s^{-1} increases the tibial shock by almost 70%. Studies examining the effect of running on different surfaces (Kim & Voloshin 1994) have produced unexpected results. Running on grass produced tibial shocks that were 25–30% higher than either asphalt or polyurethane top track. The result has been explained by the inability to anticipate the changes in the evenness of the ground underlying the grass; the body appears to stiffen in anticipation of a pos-

sible irregular landing. These results, although somewhat paradoxical, are consistent with the previously discussed data on GRF while running on grass and concrete. Thus, contrary to common belief, biomechanical research suggests that running on grass may expose the body's lower extremity joints to higher risks of degenerative damage.

Changes in the slope of the running surface also affects the shock experienced by the lower limb. Running uphill produces exponential decreases in shank acceleration, while running downhill produces exponential increases. Acceleration peaks in excess of 20 g have been measured during downhill running, which suggest that running downhill substantially increases the risk of injury to the lower extremities.

Effects of footwear

The use of appropriate footwear can result in sizeable reductions in peak shank acceleration and frequency content during running. On average, peak shank shock is some 25% lower during shod than barefoot running. Peak head shock was also reduced with the use of footwear. Both the magnitude and the frequency content of shock have been linked to the risk of degenerative joint injuries confirming the health benefits of wearing footwear to run.

In contrast to GRF studies which are unable to demonstrate a link between footwear construction and impact loads, results of acceleration studies indicate that footwear construction plays a crucial part in the reduction of impact loading during running. Because of its strategic location between the foot and the ground, the shoe midsole has attracted the attention of designers and engineers as the most likely footwear structure to regulate body shock. Peak shank shock differences ranging between 7 and 11% have been recorded for footwear that differs only in midsole construction. Other footwear features combined with midsole construction can produce even greater variation in shank shock than midsole construction alone.

Using the human pendulum to compare soft and hard midsole materials, Lafortune *et al.* (1996) reported that peak shocks were higher with the harder midsole material. In their experimental set-up, which controlled for initial impact conditions, they found that knee angle had considerable influence on the temporal and spectral features of the shock transmis-

Chapter 4

Training techniques
for successful running
performance

Historical evolution of training practices

Since the early 1900s the training and competitive practices of runners have passed through several distinct phases, most of which can be linked to either the contemporary view of training at that time, or the techniques of a successful coach credited with developing a number of world-class runners. At the turn of the century a major change in training strategy took place when runners in general, and sprinters in particular, ceased to prepare for specific races as they had in earlier days. Indeed, it was not until Britain's Harold Abrahams employed a professional coach, Sam Mussabini, in preparation for the 1924 Olympics, that the notion that runners should train systematically and specifically for an event finally regained widespread acceptance. From the 1940s up until the early 1960s several training interventions were added to the runner's training regimen, including weight training, circuit training and hill running. However, there was little understanding of how such interventions might directly improve running speed.

With the emergence of the state-supported Eastern bloc system in the 1970s, plyometric exercises, bounding, a variety of technique drills and active and passive stretching were incorporated into the training programmes of leading runners. At about this time sprinters started to employ twice-daily training routines, as well as out-of-season training. Although the pharmacological techniques employed by athletes from Eastern bloc countries were ethically wrong and in contravention of prevailing rules, the vigorous training techniques that emanated during this period have, unquestionably, been associated with improved sprint performances.

The pattern of an increased training volume for sprinters, along with the extension of the training year, is also reflected in the practices of both middle and long distance runners. In the late nineteenth century Britain's Walter George held world marks at every distance from 1 to 10 miles, and lowered the 1-mile record four times, from 4:23 1/5 in 1880 to 4:12 3/4 in 1886, this latter mark as a professional. Such performances were achieved on twice-a-day low-volume high-quality running, supplemented with callisthenics and some brisk walking. After George, another Briton, Alfred Shrubb, continued to set new records in events from 2 miles (3218 m) up to the greatest distance covered in 1 hour. Shrubb won 20 national championships between 1900 and 1904, and was the first athlete to run under 30 min for 10 000 m (29:59.4 in 1904). His 10-mile record of 50:40.6 was only broken a quarter of a century later by Paavo Nurmi of Finland (50:15 in 1928), a time that stood for a further 17 years. In contrast to his predecessors Shrubb trained heavily, running up to 80 km a week during a build-up to major races (Noakes 1992).

The success of the Czechoslovakian runner, Emil Zatopek, throughout the 1940s and 1950s was largely attributed to a combination of a huge training volume and intense interval workouts (Noakes 1992; Sandrock 1996). At various stages of his preparation between 1949 and 1954, Zatopek was running over 200 km a week (Noakes 1992). Zatopek, who won four Olympic gold medals and set 18 world records, changed the prevailing notion of how much training a distance runner could tolerate.

In the 1960s New Zealand coach, Arthur Lydiard, popularized high-volume 'marathon' training for both middle and long distance runners. Lydiard was the first coach to prescribe marked seasonal variation in training techniques, the forerunner to the modern day concepts of periodization, multi-tier training (Martin & Coe 1991) and peaking (Lydiard & Gilmour 1962). The success of Lydiard-trained runners in the 1960 and 1964 Olympiads in races from 800 m up to the marathon convinced many coaches of the benefits of high-volume training.

It was not until the 1980s that the necessity for such high-volume training, particularly for middle distance events, was questioned. At this time, the successful coach–athlete father–son partnership of Peter and Sebastian Coe was in the ascendancy. Peter Coe believed that the middle distance events, and in particular the 800 m, were 'prolonged sprints'. Coe opted for specialized event analysis, the evaluation of training programmes based on frequent monitoring and physiological testing, and long-term planning (Martin & Coe 1991). Specialized strength conditioning in the winter build-up phase, achieved through resistance and circuit training and sustained intense hill repetitions was the foundation on which more specific preparation was based. This approach resulted in 12 world records and four Olympic medals for Sebastian Coe, the only repeat winner of the 1500 m.

There is still much debate among coaches, athletes and sports scientists as to which specific training techniques best promote the physiological attributes necessary for successful running performance and constitute the optimal training programme. While a major debate centres on the issue of quality vs. quantity, it is clear that more scientific research is required to determine the unique effects of specific training procedures on the performances of well-trained runners. In the meantime it seems plausible that the best techniques for improving performance should incorporate a blend of the training techniques used by today's top runners.

Current training practices of elite runners

Sprinters

The current training methods of top sprinters have been reviewed in detail previously (see Williams & Gandy 1994). A striking feature of contemporary techniques is that although they are more comprehensive and systematic than in earlier times, they still rely heavily on many of the traditional methods practised at the turn of the last century. Indeed, there have been few scientific breakthroughs in sprint training methods. Compared to the vast body of information on distance running available to coaches, the scientific literature on sprinting is minimal. The extent to which current training practices can be scientifically validated is far from complete. Nevertheless, the current training practices of successful sprinters can be summarized as follows:
• year-round training (2–3 h·day⁻¹) often with double periodization of the competitive year;
• a gradual and progressive increase in aerobic train-

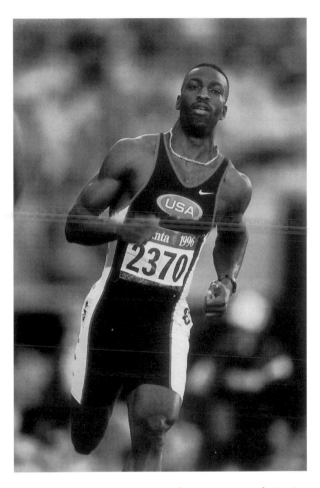

Fig. 4.1 World class sprinters employ resistance and circuit training to develop muscular strength, and a variety of forms of plyometric training and bounding to develop explosive muscle power. Michael Johnson (USA) gold medalist in the men's 200 m and 400 m at the 1996 Olympic games, Atlanta. Photo © Allsport / G.M. Prior.

ing during the general conditioning phase, including alternative modes of activity;
• extensive use of resistance and circuit training to develop muscular strength;
• plyometric training and bounding to develop explosive muscle power (Fig. 4.1);
• comprehensive use of running drills and technique work to develop neuromuscular and mechanical skill (e.g. running stadium steps);
• extensive starting practice and acceleration drills;
• uphill sprinting;
• 'overspeed' or 'supramaximal velocity' training

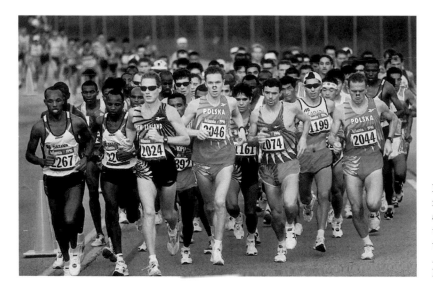

Fig. 4.2 Marathon and ultra-marathon runners undertake a high volume of aerobic conditioning, often covering up to 200 km·week⁻¹ during their base training. The men's Olympic marathon, Atlanta 1996. Photo © Allsport / G.M. Prior.

(downhill running, high-speed stationary cycling, towing or treadmill sprinting) to improve leg speed;
• use of time trials over intermediate distances;
• stretching and use of active recovery processes (massage);
• use of special dietary supplements (creatine) during periods of intensive training (see Chapter 5); and
• a long-term approach to training and competition.

Middle and long distance runners

The core components of the training systems currently employed by top middle distance and distance runners have been reviewed elsewhere (Wells & Pate 1988; Maughan 1994; Hawley & Burke 1998) and include:
• year-round training ($3-4$ h·day⁻¹) and competition with only short ($2-4$ week) breaks for active recovery;
• periodization of training;
• a high volume of aerobic conditioning (30 km·week⁻¹ for sprinters, 100 km·week⁻¹ for middle distance runners, > 200 km·week⁻¹ for long and ultra-distance runners) (Fig. 4.2);
• prolonged, steady-state running ($20-30$ km in a single session for middle distance runners, up to 50 km per session for distance and ultra-distance runners);
• a 'hard–easy' pattern to the overall organization of training;
• resistance training in the non-competitive phase;
• sustained 'tempo' or pace runs, fartlek, hill running;
• use of time trials over intermediate distances;

• stretching and mobility exercise performed after most training sessions;
• special dietary preparation before, during and after training and racing (see Chapter 5) and
• a long-term approach to training and competition.

In tracing the origins of modern-day training techniques for runners, there is little doubt that the empirical knowledge of coaches has had the greatest impact on the practices of top runners. Only recently has sports science started to make valid contributions to assist coaches in the preparation of athletes. Indeed, it could be argued that today's runners train the way they do because they and their predecessors have empirically found that certain techniques are effective. Nevertheless, analyses of the training systems of great runners from the past and present suggests that the human body responds in a predictable and uniform manner to daily training, and that such responses can be quantified. As such, there are several widely accepted scientific training principles on which all running programmes should be based.

Scientific principles of physical training

Improvements in running require long-term systematic planning, the application of appropriate training and nutrition programmes, an injury-free build-up to a competitive peak, sound tactical and pacing strategies and, on the day of a race, optimal environmental conditions. Successful performances are more likely if a runner has followed a programme based on scientific training principles than if they adopted a haphazard trial-and-error approach to their preparation. Several widely accepted training principles have evolved which are common to all running events.

Progressive overload

The principle of progressive overload states that once a runner has adapted to a specific training stimulus, the load must be increased to attain further adaptations and performance improvements. Overload can be quantified according to the volume of running (km·week^{-1}); the speed (m·s^{-1} or km·h^{-1}), load (kg lifted) or rating of perceived effort; and the frequency of running (number of training sessions per day or specified time period). The degree of adaptation to any training programme depends on the interaction between these variables and the ability of the runner to meet them.

Recovery

A training session is only beneficial if it forces the body to adapt to the stress of a particular workout. If the session is too easy, then no adaptation will occur. Conversely, if the stress of the workout (or series of workouts) is too great (performed too quickly or performed too often without adequate recovery), then performance will decline. One of the roles of the coach is to be aware of the signs and symptoms of overtraining and ensure that programmes are structured to attain the maximal physiological adaptation with the minimum risk of injury or illness (see Chapter 6).

Specificity

Any training-induced adaptation is specific to the mode of exercise performed so the closer a training routine is to the requirements of the runner's event, then the better will be the subsequent performance. For this reason, the core of any runner's training programme should reflect the desired training adaptation.

Reversibility and the loss of training-induced adaptations

Reversibility is the principle of detraining, or the loss of training-induced adaptations. Our knowledge of detraining and the retention of training adaptations

is limited to a few scientific studies, but the available evidence suggests that to minimize the loss of adaptation, runners should try to continue with the primary mode of exercise or employ alternate exercise modes which have neuromuscular recruitment patterns similar to running.

Individuality and the genetic ceiling

Although the general principles of training can be applied to runners of all abilities, the magnitude of adaptation to a particular workout is likely to vary considerably between runners. The coach must evaluate the physiological requirements of a runner's event and then assess each athlete's ability to meet those demands. Genetic factors, for example, can be responsible for up to 80% of the variability in the magnitude of adaptation to a training stimulus, and subsequent performance (for review see Bouchard *et al.* 1992).

Structure of training programmes

A prerequisite for successful performance is planning the structure of a runner's training programme. Periodization refers to the organization of a runner's training system into distinct phases. Such periodization must take into consideration a runner's immediate (weeks), medium (months) and long-term (years) competition objectives. During each phase, primary emphasis is given to the development of one (or more) physiological objectives. Most training cycles normally fit into a single periodized year, but with the advent of year-round competition (the indoor circuit, northern and southern hemisphere seasons), many international runners will have to 'double-periodize' their training cycles.

The phases (or macrocycles) of any training programme for runners can be broadly split into four main categories:
1 the conditioning or general preparatory phase;
2 the transition or competition preparation phase;
3 the competition phase, including taper and;
4 the recovery phase.

Conditioning or general preparatory phase

This phase (or mesocycle) typically lasts 8–12 weeks for high school or Masters runners and up to 6 months for an international athlete. In the case of a double-periodized year, each phase of the training cycle will be reduced accordingly. The primary aim of this phase of training is to provide a base of general conditioning on which further, more intense training can be undertaken. The primary physiological benefits of this phase of training have been detailed previously (Wells & Pate 1988).

One of the most important goals of the general preparatory phase is to condition the skeletal system, particularly the supporting muscle structures, to withstand the trauma associated with the repeated high ground reaction forces encountered while running (see Chapter 3). During this phase of training the volume of work is high and the magnitude of adaptation is likely to be greatest when the runner's weekly training load is just below that threshold that would eventually overextend the athlete and lead to staleness and fatigue. Depending on the ability of the runner, the frequency of training should be between 6 and 12 sessions a week. Most of these workouts will be spent running, with attention to technical aspects of an athlete's event. Both sprinters and distance runners often include uphill running, weight and circuit training, plyometrics and stretching routines in addition to their general running programme. Some runners employ alternative training modes, such as cycling, deep-water running or swimming during this phase.

Transition or competition preparation phase

The transition phase should last 4–8 weeks, depending on the length of the subsequent competition phase. The primary aim of this phase of training is to expose the various physiological power systems to sustained intense running at velocities close to, or faster than, planned race pace, thereby improving the athlete's resistance to fatigue. The results of one scientific investigation support such an approach. Acevedo and Goldfarb (1989) studied seven trained distance runners with a mean maximal oxygen uptake ($\dot{V}O_{2max}$) of 65.5 ml·kg^{-1}·min^{-1}, who replaced a portion of their weekly running with transition workouts at speeds equal to or slightly faster than their (current) 10-km race pace. Runners completed the transition sessions on Monday, Wednesday and Friday while continuing to cover 8–20 km·day^{-1} on the other days of the week. After 8 weeks of running at an increased intensity for three sessions a week, 10-km race time improved an average of *c.* 3%, from 35:27 to 34:24.

This was accomplished despite the absence of any change in the runner's $\dot{V}O_{2max}$ after the intensified training period, suggesting that distance runners who increase their training intensity can subsequently race at a higher percentage of their aerobic power.

The shift from general conditioning to the transition or competition preparation phase is also facilitated by the introduction of time trials over a variety of intermediate race distances which help to develop a runner's pace judgement. Performance tests (described later in this chapter) can also be employed. There is a slight decrease in the total volume of training, with a corresponding increase in more specific conditioning work, particularly drills, starting practice and acceleration runs for the sprinter. During the competition preparation phase no emphasis should be placed on alternative training modes. Despite recommendations from some exercise physiologists that training prescription during this phase of training should be based on specific blood lactate concentrations (i.e. 4 mmol·l^{-1}), there is no scientific evidence to support such claims. However, continuous training at individually prescribed heart rates might be a useful adjunct for monitoring the intensity of workouts.

Competition phase (including taper)

This entire phase can last from 2 to 4 months depending on the ability level of the runner. The primary aim of this phase of training is to prepare the runner for several major competitive peaks within the cycle. There is a further decrease in the volume of training to facilitate adequate recovery between training sessions and races. The principal emphasis for middle distance and distance runners is the inclusion of workbouts undertaken at speeds faster than planned race pace. Such 'speedwork' entails intense, short duration running with near complete (several minutes) recovery. For sprinters, this phase incorporates supramaximal efforts at distances less than planned competition distance. In the taper, weight and circuit training and plyometric exercise are stopped. During the 3–5 days prior to a major race, runners should reduce the volume of training so that it is almost zero in the 2–3 days before the race. This reduction in training volume, necessary for an effective taper, should not be achieved at the expense of a big drop-off in the number of training sessions undertaken; the runner should not reduce training *frequency* by more than 30% than is normal for this phase of training.

The results of several studies show that a taper improves middle distance running performance by *c.* 3% (Shepley *et al.* 1992; Houmard *et al.* 1994). The mechanisms responsible for such an enhancement include an elevation in resting muscle glycogen content, an increase in total blood volume, enhanced muscle oxidative enzyme activity and improved running economy. There may also be subtle, but physiologically important, changes in muscle contractile function with the taper which allow the runner to generate greater peak forces (sprinting) and sustain faster maximal running velocities (middle distance and distance events), possibly by higher motor unit activation.

Recovery phase

This phase should last between 4 and 6 weeks, depending on the periodization of the runner's year and their level of ability. The primary aim of this phase of training is to allow the athlete an extended period of recuperation, physically and psychologically, from the preceding season. The presence of any chronic injury and its complete rehabilitation should be addressed. To this end, stretching and other means of recovery (massage, whirlpool, etc.) can be employed. Depending on the length of the preceding competition phase, the runner may need a period of complete inactivity before embarking on a period of 'active rest' where training is gradually resumed. For the coach, this phase permits an evaluation of training and racing from the previous season, and the revision of future goals based on the runner's progress to date.

Training programmes for running

Training for running can be defined as a systematic planned programme of physical preparation for the sole purpose of improving performance. Intuitively, the perfect training regimen for the enhancement of running performance should incorporate most of the training techniques currently practised by top runners. Such logic, however, ignores the principle of individuality and the genetic component of performance; those runners who are capable of exceptional performances are not only genetically well endowed, but can also optimize these traits through appropriate training. Comprehensive details of training

programmes for sprinters, middle and long distance runners for each phase of the training cycle and for runners of different ability levels are beyond the scope of this chapter. Instead, examples of training regimens for runners from a variety of events have been provided. In conjunction with the data on the energetics of running (see Chapters 1 and 2) and the overview of the scientific principles of physical training and the structure of training programmes, it is hoped that the schedules that follow will provide a framework on which coaches can construct individualized programmes for their runners.

Sprinters

Table 4.1 details the training guidelines constructed by Williams and Gandy (1994) for 100–200 m sprinters who have two competitive seasons each year (double periodization). They provide an excellent framework on which the fundamentals of a training programme should be based. For simplicity they have been divided into eight phases encompassing general preparation, competition preparation and a transition period between seasons.

Middle distance runners

One of the features of successful runners is a long-term outlook to training and racing. The schedules detailed are those of Noureddine Morceli (Morocco) (Table 4.2) and Sebastian Coe (Great Britain) (Table 4.3), both winners of the Olympic 1500 m title and world record holders for the mile (1609 m). They illustrate the principle of progressive development and planning towards long-term competition goals. In 1973, aged 16, Sebastian Coe won the English Schools 3000 m in 8:40.2 and also ran 3:55 for the 1500 m. In 1975 he was third in the European Junior Championships running 3:45.2 for the 1500 m and the following year broke 4:00 min for the mile for the first time (3:58.3). By 1978, aged 21, Coe had broken the UK 800-m record (1:43.97). World records in the 800 m (1:42.33), 1500 m (3:32.03) and 1 mile (3:48.95) followed in 1979. In 1986, at the age of 29, Coe ran a lifetime best of 3:29.77 for the 1500 m and, at the age of 32, was still capable of 1:43.38 for 800 m.

Like Coe, Noureddine Morceli's athletic progression was gradual. As late as 1990, Morceli was still training only once a day, yet was still capable of running a

Table 4.1 Training guidelines for 100–200 m sprinters. Reproduced with permission from Williams and Gandy (1994)

Phase 1: General preparation I (10–12 weeks)
1 Build up to full training routine
2 All round conditioning (weights, circuits, stretching) and alternative training methods (running in water, ergometer cycling)
3 Technical aspects of sprinting at 80% of max. effort
4 Aerobic work (3–5 km runs) and fartlek/track work (e.g. 6 × 200 m with 200 m jog recovery)

Phase 2: Competition preparation I (4 weeks)
1 Maintain full training programme with more specific conditioning work
2 Development of technique drills and starting practice (e.g. 5–8 reps up to 40 m with 3–5 min recovery)
3 Performance tests

Phase 3: Indoor competitions (4–8 weeks)
1 Reduction in training routine to promote recovery and sharpness
2 Competition-specific technical work (acceleration and max. speed sessions)

Phase 4: General preparation II (6–8 weeks)
As for phase 1 but less aerobic work and more volume in track sessions (e.g. 6 × 300 m with 500 m jog recovery and/or sets of 4 × 30, 4 × 40, 4 × 50, 4 × 60, 4 × 50, 4 × 40, 4 × 30 m with 90 s recovery)

Phase 5: Competition preparation II (4–5 weeks)
1 Speed endurance track sessions (e.g. 2–4 sets of 3–4 reps of 90–150 m with 90–120 s between runs and 5–10 min between sets)
2 Greater emphasis on speed (starting practice, technique running)
3 Performance testing and time trials

Phase 6: Outdoor competition I (4 weeks)
1 Similar to phase 3 but including an enhanced speed–endurance component
2 Technical aspects of sprinting (e.g. start, accelerations, form)
3 Conduct 3–5 competitions as time trials

Phase 7: Outdoor competition II (8–12 weeks)
1 Participate in 10–15 planned races aiming at personal best performances in key races
2 Training scheduled around competition and emphasis on speed and sharpness

Phase 8: Transition period (4–6 weeks)
1 Rest and recovery from previous season
2 Evaluation of training and racing and establish future plans and goals

Table 4.2 Conditioning programme for Noureddine Morceli for the 1990 track season. Reproduced with permission from Sandrock (1996)

Monday	(p.m.)	Road run (1 h)
		Steady pace, hard. Finish run at track with some easy strides
Tuesday	(p.m.)	Very easy jog (1 h)
		Pace 12 km·h⁻¹
Wednesday	(p.m.)	Track session
		Warm-up jog and strides, then:
		10–12 × 400 m 'fast and relaxed'. The recovery was often 110 m jog, but when preparing for the 5000 m this was reduced to 55 m.
		Warm-down jog
Thursday	(p.m.)	Same as Tuesday
Friday	(p.m.)	Fartlek session (1 h)
		Undertaken on golf course, undulating
Saturday	(p.m.)	Easy day or rest
Sunday	(a.m.)	Long run (60–90 min)
		Relaxed pace (15 km·h⁻¹)

3:55.83 mile and 13:25.2 for the 5000 m. He did not start running twice a day until late in 1991, his training load having been gradually increased over a 3-year period. In 1991 he clocked 3:31.2 for 1500 m and also won the World Championships in Tokyo (3:32.84). Despite a disappointing 1992 Olympics (Morceli was placed seventh in the 1500 m in a slow tactical race), that year he broke the world 1500 m record, running 3:28.86. Late in 1993 he became the first runner to break 3:45 for the mile (3:44.39) and three years later won the Olympic gold medal in the 1500 m. The programme outlined in Table 4.2 is Morceli's conditioning phase for the 1990 track season.

The training schedule in Table 4.3 for Coe illustrates the shift in emphasis from volume to quality running in the immediate build-up to a competition. The programme given is a week in mid-July immediately prior to the 1984 Olympics. Coe, who was doubling in the 800 and 1500 m, had seven races in 9 days which he used as part of his taper and competition preparation. For the 5 weeks leading up to the Olympics, Coe's training volume totalled 61, 58, 50, 38 and 27 km·week⁻¹.

Table 4.3 Pre-Olympic training programme for Sebastian Coe, 1984. Reproduced with permission from Sandrock (1996)

Monday	(a.m.)	Tempo running Warm-up jog and strides, then: 6 × 800 m in 2 min with 3 min recovery. Warm-down 800 m at 16 km·h⁻¹ pace and easy jogging
	(p.m.)	Easy run (6–7 km)
Tuesday	(a.m.)	Easy run (8 km)
	(p.m.)	Warm-up jog and strides, then: 10 × 100 m steady acceleration to 60 m, maximum speed to 80 m, float last 20 m. Walk back recovery. Warm-down jog
Wednesday	(a.m.)	Warm-up jog and strides, then: 6 × 300 m in 41 s with 3 min jog recovery. Warm-down jog
	(p.m.)	Easy run (6–7 km)
Thursday	(a.m.)	Track session (speedwork) Warm-up jog and strides, then: 20 × 200 m in 27–28 s with 90 s recovery. Warm-down jog
	(p.m.)	Easy run (8 km)
Friday	(p.m.)	Track session Warm-up jog and strides, then: 'up-the-clock' session. 100,110,120,130,140,150,140,130, 120,110,100 m fast and relaxed sprints with jog back recovery. Warm-down jog
Saturday	(p.m.)	Endurance run/fartlek (10–11 km)

Table 4.4 Pre-marathon training programme for Tegla Laroupe. Reproduced with permission from Tanser (1997)

Monday	(a.m.)	Easy run (60 min) Pace 15 km·h⁻¹
	(p.m.)	Easy run (60 min) Pace 15 km·h⁻¹
Tuesday	(a.m.)	Easy run (90 min)
Wednesday	(a.m.)	Easy run (60–120 min)
	(p.m.)	Easy run (60 min)
Thursday	(a.m.)	Interval training (track or flat terrain) Warm-up jog, then: 3 × 3 km at marathon pace (3 : 18 min·km⁻¹) with 2 min jog recovery, *or* 15 × 1 km at faster than race pace with 'minimal' recovery
	(p.m.)	Easy run (90 min)
Friday	(a.m.)	Easy run (75 min)
	(p.m.)	Jogging
Saturday	(a.m.)	Long run (150 min)
Sunday	(a.m.)	Tempo run (90 min) First hour easy, then last 30 min hard

Long distance runners

In the last decade, the accomplishments of several of the African nations in long distance running has been phenomenal. African runners, or runners born in Africa and now competing for other nations, currently hold the men's world records for every track distance from 800 m up to 10 000 m. In the 1997 world rankings, African runners held 39 out of 50 (78%) of the top 10 fastest times in all men's Olympic events from 800 to 10 000 m. Whatever the reason for such dominance, the training programmes reported for African runners bear a strong resemblance to the systems outlined above and currently employed by top distance runners from many other nations. Perhaps the only

differences are the speed of the majority of running sessions and the complete lack of weight or circuit training.

Although Kenyan men have dominated distance running since the early 1990s, only recently have their women begun to make a significant impact on the world scene. One runner in particular, Tegla Laroupe, has spearheaded the Kenyan women's challenge. Laroupe ran middle distances as a junior, gradually moving up to the longer races. Winning the New York marathon at her first attempt in 1994, and subsequently in 1995, Laroupe broke the world best for this distance in 1998 (2:20:47), a record that had stood since 1985. Laroupe takes a 3-month build-up to a major marathon and includes under-distance track races as part of her speedwork and taper. After racing a marathon, she takes 2–4 weeks rest and active recovery before embarking on another conditioning phase. The schedule in Table 4.4 is a typical week during the build-up to a marathon. The volume is high (25–30 km·day⁻¹) with most of the runs on hilly trails, at an altitude of between 1300 and 2700 m.

Ultra-distance runners

Ultra-distance races are categorized as being longer than the standard marathon (42.2 km) up to furthest distance a runner can cover in 24 h. In recent years there has been a growing participation in ultra-distance events by a number of top long distance runners. One of the most successful runners is the Scotsman, Donald Ritchie, whose athletic career has extended over a quarter of a century and includes nine world best times for track distances from 50 km up to 200 km. At the age of 54 he was still fast enough to gain selection for the British national team to contest the European 100 km championships and the European 24 h race.

Ritchie, who is self-coached, takes a 10-week build-up to major races, and gradually increases his base mileage from about 170 km·week⁻¹ up to a high of 260 km·week⁻¹. When training he emphasizes a high carbohydrate diet with little fibre and meat. Massage is also an important part of the recovery process, especially during ultra-distance races. A normal training regimen would involve running twice each day, Monday to Friday, with single runs on Saturday and Sunday. According to Ritchie, the key to successful racing over ultra-distances are the once-a-week long run of at least 2 hours' duration. Most of Ritchie's training is accomplished at paces of 16 km·h⁻¹ or faster which, considering the volume, is formidable and similar to many middle distance and distance runners. Nearly all of his training is done alone. The schedule in Table 4.5 is the 2-week period before a major race, encompassing the taper phase.

Performance tests for runners

It has become commonplace for coaches to incorporate some measure of performance testing into the training programmes of their athletes. Such testing, when undertaken regularly over several seasons, can provide important information about the physiological status of an individual runner, as well as giving a measure of progress towards specified long- and short-term goals. There are many valid and reliable laboratory-based tests for runners which have been reviewed elsewhere (Maud & Foster 1995; Hawley 1999). Only information about field-based performance tests is provided here.

Table 4.5 Two-week training programme before a major race for Donald Ritchie (from Ritchie 1993)

Monday	(a.m.)	13 km
Tuesday	(p.m.)	13 km
Wednesday	(a.m.)	22 km
	(p.m.)	22 km
Thursday	(a.m.)	22 km
	(p.m.)	27 km
		13 km 'hard'
Friday	(a.m.)	27 km
	(p.m.)	20 km
Saturday		No training
Sunday		50 km in 3.00.48
Monday	(p.m.)	28 km
Tuesday	(a.m.)	22 km
	(p.m.)	14 km
Wednesday	(a.m.)	22 km
	(p.m.)	22 km
Thursday	(a.m.)	22 km
	(p.m.)	14 km then 5–6 km time trial
Friday		No training
Saturday		No training
Sunday		Race: London to Brighton (53.5 miles/ 85.6 km)
		Time: 5:13.02
		First position, fastest ever average speed for this event

Table 4.6 displays performance standards for a variety of skills for sprinters with target race times for the 100 m ranging from 10.70 to 10.00 s. It is clear that in order to attain several of the criteria listed, a sprinter must posses a high peak running velocity, a high degree of explosive muscle power for rapid acceleration, coordination and skill. For middle distance runners, the Kosmin test (Table 4.7) has been devised to project a runner's current 800 m race time from the total distance a runner can cover during two maximal 60 s efforts with a recovery interval of 3 min. Such a test is often preferred by middle distance runners compared to a time trial over their competitive race distance.

The Kosmin test can also provide a coach with additional physiological information that, for example, may not be apparent from a tactically run race won in

Table 4.6 Performance standards for 100-m sprinters. Reproduced with permission from Tabatschnik (1983)

Skill	Target time for the 100 m			
	10.70 s	10.50 s	10.20 s	10.00 s
Sprint 30 m, crouch start (s)	4.1–4.2	4.0–4.1	3.8–3.9	3.7–3.8
Sprint 30 m (flying start)	2.9–3.0	2.8–2.9	2.75–2.80	2.7
Peak sprint velocity (m·s⁻¹)	10.86	11.11	11.62	11.90
Sprint 150 m (s)	15.7	15.2	14.8	14.7
Sprint 300 m (s)	35.2–36.2	34.0–35.0	32.4–33.2	31.0–32.4
Standing long jump (m)	2.85–2.90	2.90–3.00	3.00–3.10	3.00–3.10
Sanding triple jump (m)	8.60–8.80	8.90–9.20	9.30–10.00	9.30–10.00
10 hops (standing start) (m)	33–34	34–35	35–36	35–36

a slow time. An athlete who covers 450 m in the first 60 s effort, for example, followed by 400 m in the second run has covered a total distance of 850 m for a predicted race time of 1:56.2 for 800 m (see Table 4.7). However, such a large drop-off (> 10%) in the distance of the second 60 s effort suggests that this runner would be well advised to undertake more speed–endurance training before they race successfully.

Table 4.8 provides several formulae for runners wishing to predict their potential performance at a distance at which they have not recently competed, from a recent race performance over a different distance.

Finally, Table 4.9 displays several performance standards for running distances from 100 m up to 10 000 m, as well as some ancillary skills for young male long distance runners.

All performance testing should provide the coach with rapid meaningful practical data on which to fine-tune a runner's training programme. In the final analysis, the results obtained from either laboratory or field testing should be used to complement the observations of a coach and neither should be considered a replacement for the other. In the future, it would be helpful for the exercise physiologist to have a complete battery of tests for runners of different abilities, competing over the range of running distances. There is also a scarcity of data pertaining to the female runner.

Specialized training strategies

Altitude training

Many coaches firmly believe that preparation for a major sea level competition is incomplete unless a runner has undertaken a period of altitude training. Indeed, the prevailing opinion amongst sports practitioners is that altitude training can improve the sea level performance of *any* runner irrespective of their event. While the physiological adaptations from altitude training have been well documented (Wolski *et al*. 1996), the effects on running performance were, until recently, not so clear.

There are three basic approaches to altitude training for runners who normally reside at sea level. The traditional strategy has been short-term (3–4 weeks) constant exposure to an altitude of 2000–3000 m. A second technique is several intermittent (1–2 weeks) exposures to altitude, separated by periods (2–3 weeks) of sea level training. Finally, the altitude training strategy that might allow the runner the best of both worlds would be to live at altitude and to train at sea level ('live high, train low'). Such an approach should enable the runner to acquire the physiological advantages of constant altitude acclimatization, without experiencing the associated drop-off in training intensity typically associated with hypoxic exercise. Evidence from one recent study tends to support such a hypothesis.

Table 4.7 The Kosmin test to predict current 800 m race time from the distance covered in 2 × 60 s runs

Total distance covered in 2 × 60 s (m)	Projected 800 m race time (min:s)
805	2:01.6
810	2:01.0
815	2:00.4
820	1:59.8
825	1:59.2
830	1:58.6
835	1:58.0
840	1:57.4
845	1:56.8
850	1:50.2
855	1:55.7
860	1:55.1
865	1:54.5
870	1:53.9
875	1:53.5
880	1:52.7
885	1:52.1
890	1:51.3
895	1:50.9
900	1:50.3
905	1:49.7
910	1:49.1
915	1:48.5
920	1:47.9
925	1:47.3
930	1:46.6
935	1:46.0
940	1:45.4
945	1:44.8
950	1:44.2

The runner is allowed 180 s recovery between the two 60 s efforts.

Table 4.8 Formulae for predicting potential race times over a number of distances from recent performance times. Reproduced with permission from Martin and Coe (1991)

Marathon = 4.76 Y		
10 000 m = Y	10 000 m = 2.1 Y	
5000 m = 0.48 Y	*5000 m = Y*	5000 m = 3.63 Y
3000 m = 0.28 Y	3000 m = 0.58 Y	3000 m = 2.15 Y
1500 m = 0.13 Y	1500 m = 0.27 Y	*1500 m = Y*
	800 m = 0.13 Y	800 m = 0.48 Y
	400 m = 0.66 Y	400 m = 0.22 Y

The performance distance in italics is the runner's specialist distance.

altitude or sea level training camps. After 4 weeks of specialized training all runners were retested.

Both high–high and high–low training significantly improved the runner's red cell mass (12%), haemoglobin concentration (9%) and $\dot{V}_{O_{2max}}$ (5%), whereas there was no change in any of these variables for the low–low group. However, only the high–low group were able to transfer these physiological adaptations into an improved maximum running speed (7% faster) and a quicker 5000 m time (3.6% faster). Such improvements were, presumably, brought about by the maintenance of near sea level training velocities in the high–low compared to the high–high runners. These results support the use of the high–low strategy for altitude acclimatization for improvements in sea level performance in middle distance running events lasting 15–20 min (Levine & Stray-Gundersen 1997).

To date, there is no scientific evidence that altitude training improves sprint running, although it is feasible that muscle buffering capacity might be altered by such an intervention. In theory, improved muscle buffering capacity ought to improve performances of those runners whose event relies predominantly on the anaerobic power systems, such as the sprints and middle distance races. If altitude training is to be employed as part of a runner's competition preparation, coaches should be aware that not all athletes will respond similarly to such exposure. Furthermore, training at elevations > 3500 m results in a high incidence of altitude sickness, accompanied by a significant drop in aerobic power and training intensity. Therefore, the recommended elevation for altitude training is between 2200 and 2500 m (Wolski *et al.* 1996).

The effects of either living at moderate altitude (2500 m) and training at low (1250 m) altitude (high–low); living and training at moderate (2500 m) altitude (high–high); or living and training at sea level (low–low), on 5000 m time were investigated in 39 competitive middle distance runners (Levine & Stray-Gundersen 1997). All runners undertook 6 weeks of supervised sea level training then ran a 5000 m time trial as well as performing a variety of laboratory tests before being randomly assigned to one of the three

Table 4.9 Suggested performance standards for running and some ancillary skills for young male long distance runners. Reproduced with permission from Suslov and Nikitushkin (1995)

Task	Under 16 years (Category I)	Under 16 years (Category II)	Under 18 years (Category I)	Under 18 years (Category II)
100 m sprint (s)	13.3	13.6	12.4	12.9
400 m sprint (s)	60.0	61.5	55.0	58.5
800 m run (min:s)	2:12.0	2:15.0	2:03	2:08
1000 m run (min:s)	2:55.0	2:59.0	2:43.5	2:50.0
1500 m run (min:s)	4:30.0	4:30.0	4:12.0	4:26.0
3000 m run (min:s)	9:30.0	9:43.0	8:52.0	9:16.0
5000 m run (min:s)	16:40.0	17:40.0	15:30.0	16:10.0
10 000 m run (min:s)	35:27	36:00	33:00	34:25
Standing long jump (m)	2.40	2.35	2.60	2.50
Standing triple jump (m)	7.25	7.10	7.80	7.50
Standing 10 jumps (m)	24.50	24.00	26.30	25.25

Pacing

Given the importance of tactics and pacing on running events lasting longer than a few seconds, there has been very little scientific study of how different pacing strategies might influence the outcome of competitive middle and long distance races. It is generally believed that after an initial acceleration phase, 'even pace' running leads to the fastest overall times in middle and long distance races. Such a premise is based on limited physiological and experimental data collected 40 years ago (for review see Foster *et al.* 1994). Yet analyses of pacing strategies of runners during competition reveal that all athletes show a significant deceleration in the second half of a race (Foster *et al.* 1994; van Ingen Schenau *et al.* 1994). The question arises as to what extent a runner might be able to improve performance if the optimal pacing strategy was adopted.

For sprinting no such strategy is necessary; a maximal effort from the start is required (Fig. 4.3), even if these tactics cause a significant reduction in running velocity towards the end of a race (see Chapter 1; van Ingen Schenau *et al.* 1994). World class sprinters must be able to generate instantaneous peak power outputs of > 3000 W (men) and > 1500 W (women) when accelerating from the starting blocks (van Ingen Schenau *et al.* 1994) in order to attain maximal run-

ning speeds of > 11.5 m·s^{-1} (males) and > 10.0 m·s^{-1} (females). Elite sprinters are not only able to achieve high running velocities, but also maintain these velocities longer throughout a race. Table 4.10 shows that the first four finishers at the 1991 World Athletic Championships were not only capable of reaching high peak sprinting speeds, but were also able to sustain such speeds right up to the final stages of the race.

For sprinters of various performance levels, the differences in the initial acceleration phase during a 100-m sprint are relatively small, while the differences in maximal running velocity are much more pronounced (van Ingen Schenau *et al.* 1994). This means that techniques such as 'overspeed' or 'supramaximal velocity training' aimed at increasing stride rate and speed should be incorporated into a sprinter's training regimen.

When running events last longer than 80 s, even-paced strategies should be adopted (Foster *et al.* 1994; van Ingen Schenau *et al.* 1994). The closer a runner can come to achieving 'even splits' for the first and second half of a race, the better the final performance. Data from the 1988 Olympic 800-m finals reveal that in both men's and women's races, all runners had slower second laps than first (8.85 and 7.26% slower, respectively), but that the race winners had the smallest drop-off during the second half of the race (2.54%). Runners should aim to practise variations in pacing

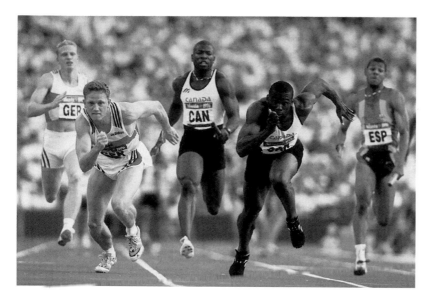

Fig. 4.3 World class sprinters must be able to generate high instantaneous peak power outputs when either accelerating from the starting blocks or during the exchange in a relay race, in order to attain maximal running speeds. The men's 4 × 100 m Olympic sprint relay final, Atlanta 1996. Canada won the gold medal. Photo © Allsport / G. Mortimore.

Table 4.10 Breakdown of the average running velocities for the fastest four finishers in the men's 100-m final at the 1991 World Athletic Championships. Data from Ae and Suzuki (1992)

Elapsed distance (m)	Carl Lewis (m·s⁻¹)	Leroy Burrell (m·s⁻¹)	Dennis Mitchell (m·s⁻¹)	Linford Christie (m·s⁻¹)
10	5.31	5.46	5.56	5.41
20	9.26	9.43	9.35	9.43
30	10.87	10.99	10.75	10.87
40	11.24	11.36	11.36	11.24
50	11.90	11.49	11.49	*11.76*
60	11.76	11.63	11.49	11.63
70	11.90	11.49	*11.63*	11.63
80	*12.05*	*11.90*	*11.63*	*11.76*
90	11.49	11.24	11.36	11.11
100	11.63	11.49	11.24	11.36
Final time (s)	9.86	9.88	9.91	9.92

The numbers in italics show the race segment at which each runner attained peak velocity.

strategy during time trials in training or in minor competitions.

Conclusions

Training is not, and is unlikely ever to be, a purely scientific endeavour. Our current knowledge of the most appropriate training practices for running have evolved through the observations and experiences of many coaches and their athletes, and not because of any revolutionary scientific breakthroughs arising from laboratory-based investigations by sports scientists. While many runners undertake resistance and circuit training, stretching, uphill and downhill running, plyometrics and other activities, there is currently little scientific evidence that such practices are of direct benefit to running performance. Indeed, the extent to which present-day training methods have been scientifically substantiated is far from complete. For example, there is a clear need for further investigations into precompetition taper strategies for different running events. More applied research is urgently needed to establish the 'science of training' and provide a body of knowledge which complements the field-based observations of coaches.

References

Acevedo, E.O. & Goldfarb, A.H. (1989) Increased training intensity effects on plasma lactate, ventilatory threshold, and endurance. *Medicine and Science in Sports and Exercise* **21**, 563–568.

Ae, M. & Suzuki, M. (1992) The men's 100 metres. *New Studies in Athletics* **7**, 47–52.

Bouchard, C., Dionne, F.T., Simoneau, J.A. & Boulay, M.R. (1992) Genetics of aerobic and anaerobic performances. In: *Exercise and Sports Science Reviews*, Vol. 20, (ed. J.O. Holloszy), pp. 27–58. Williams & Wilkins, Baltimore.

Foster, C., Schrager, M., Snyder, A.C. & Thompson, N.N. (1994) Pacing strategy and athletic performance. *Sports Medicine* **17**, 77–85.

Hawley, J.A. (1999) Laboratory and field tests of athletic potential and performance. In: *Basic and Applied Science for Sports Medicine* (ed. R.J. Maughan), pp. 312–315. Butterworth–Heinemann, Oxford.

Hawley, J.A. & Burke, L.M. (1998) *Peak Performance: Training and Nutritional Strategies for Sport*. Allen and Unwin, Sydney.

Houmard, J.A., Scott, B.K., Justice, C.L. & Chenier, T.C. (1994) The effects of taper on performance in distance runners. *Medicine and Science in Sports and Exercise* **26**, 624–631.

Levine, B.D. & Stray-Gundersen, J. (1997) 'Living high–training low': effect of moderate-altitude acclimatization with low-altitude training on performance. *Journal of Applied Physiology* **83**, 102–112.

Lydiard, A. & Gilmour, G. (1962) *Run to the Top*. A.H. & A. Reed, Wellington.

Martin, D.E. & Coe, P.N. (1991) *Training Distance Runners*. Leisure Press, Champaign, Illinois.

Maud, P.J. & Foster, C. (1995) *Physiological Assessment of Human Fitness*. Human Kinetics, Champaign, Illinois.

Maughan, R.J. (1994) Physiology and nutrition for middle distance and long distance running. In: *Perspectives in Exercise Science and Sports Medicine*, Vol. 7. *Physiology and Nutrition in Competitive Sport*, (eds D.R. Lamb, H. Knuttgen & R. Murray), pp. 329–371. Cooper Publishing, Carmel, Indianapolis.

Noakes, T.D. (1992) *Lore of Running*, 3rd edn, pp. 128–270. Oxford University Press, Cape Town.

Ritchie, D. (1993) Training. In: *Training for Ultras*, (ed. A. Milroy), 2nd edn, pp. 29–38. Road Runners Club, Surrey.

Sandrock, M. (1996) *Running with the Legends: Training and Racing Insights from 21 Great Runners*. Human Kinetics, Champaign, Illinois.

Shepley, B., MacDougall, J.D., Cipriano, N. *et al.* (1992) Physiological effects of tapering in highly trained athletes. *Journal of Applied Physiology* **72**, 706–711.

Suslov, F. & Nikitushkin, V. (1995) What a coach should take into account in the preparation of young runners. In: *Long Distances: Contemporary Theory, Technique and Training* (ed. J. Jarver), pp. 97–99. Track and Field News, Mountain View, California.

Tabatschnik, B. (1983) Looking for 100-m speed. *Modern Athlete and Coach* **9**, 14–16.

Tanser, T. (1997) *Train Hard, Win Easy: the Kenyan Way*, p. 175. Track and Field News Press, Mountain View, California.

Van Ingen Schenau, G.J., de Koning, J.J. & de Groot, G. (1994) Optimisation of sprinting performance in running, cycling and speed skating. *Sports Medicine* **17**, 259–275.

Wells, C.L. & Pate, R.R. (1988) Training for performance of prolonged exercise. In: *Perspectives in Exercise Science and Sports Medicine*, Vol. 1. *Prolonged Exercise* (eds D.R. Lamb & R. Murray), pp. 357–391. Benchmark Press, Carmel, Indianapolis.

Williams, C. & Gandy, G. (1994) Physiology and nutrition for sprinting. In: *Perspectives in Exercise Science and Sports Medicine*, Vol. 7. *Physiology and Nutrition for Competitive Sport*, (eds D.R. Lamb, H.G. Knuttgen & R. Murray), pp. 55–98. Cooper Publishing Group, Carmel, Indiana.

Wolski, L.A., McKenzie, D.C. & Wenger, H.A. (1996) Altitude training for improvements in sea level performance: is there scientific evidence of benefit? *Sports Medicine* **22**, 251–263.

Recommended reading

Hawley, J.A. & Burke, L.M. (1998) *Peak Performance: Training and Nutritional Strategies for Sport*. Allen and Unwin, Sydney.

Maughan, R.J. (1994) Physiology and nutrition for middle distance and long distance running. In: *Perspectives in Exercise Science and Sports Medicine*, Vol. 7. *Physiology and Nutrition in Competitive Sport*, (eds D.R. Lamb, H. Knuttgen & R. Murray), pp. 329–371. Cooper Publishing, Carmel, Indianapolis.

Noakes, T.D. (1992) *Lore of Running*, 3rd edn. Oxford University Press, Cape Town.

Sandrock, M. (1996) *Running with the Legends: Training and Racing Insights from 21 Great Runners*. Human Kinetics, Champaign, Illinois.

Wells, C.L. & Pate, R.R. (1988) Training for performance of prolonged exercise. In: *Perspectives in Exercise Science and Sports Medicine*, Vol. 1. *Prolonged Exercise* (eds D.R. Lamb & R. Murray), pp. 357–391. Benchmark Press, Carmel, Indianapolis.

Chapter 5

Nutrition for runners

Despite the simplicity of running, the sport is endowed with a rich history and culture. Diet has played a key part in the preparation of runners throughout the ages, although it is apparent that fad and folklore are often involved and that scientific beliefs have changed over time. Much of the development of modern exercise science since the 1960s has been inspired by long distance running. Indeed, the running boom of the 1970s and 1980s first brought sports science to the 'man in the street'. Today millions of recreational runners worldwide seek nutritional and training strategies in order to enhance their performance. For a few elite runners, professional competition promises the rewards of fame and fortune for exceptional performance.

In competitive running there are three major classes of events, based on the unique physiological and nutritional characteristics they encompass. These classifications have been outlined in the previous chapters. This purpose of this chapter will be to describe the nutritional considerations and strategies for running events up to the marathon distance (42.2 km). Attention will be given to five major areas of nutrition:

1 general considerations for training nutrition;
2 strategies for nutrition before and during competitive events;
3 postexercise nutritional recovery strategies;
4 nutritional supplements; and
5 nutritional considerations for the travelling runner.

In each section the principles of sports nutrition based on the physiological requirements of the different categories of running will be discussed. In addition, common issues related to the conversion of guidelines into real life practice will be noted.

Training diet

The goal of any training programme is to prepare runners to perform at their best during major competitions (see Chapter 4). Whatever the running distance, nutrition plays a substantial part in the optimization of those factors that will enable an athlete to face the start line in the best possible condition. Everyday eating patterns must supply the runner with the fuel and nutrients needed to optimize their performance during training sessions, and also to recover quickly afterwards. The runner must also eat to stay in good health. Special strategies of food and fluid intake before, during and after a training session may help to reduce fatigue and enhance subsequent performance. These strategies will often be important in the competition setting, but must be practised and fine-tuned during training so that successful methods can be identified.

Achieving ideal body physique

Physique plays a part in the performance of many sports, and running is no exception: elite runners typically display the optimal physical characteristics for their event (see Chapters 1 and 2). This is largely the result of genetic factors that have helped to determine the runner's pursuits, along with the conditioning effects of nutrition and training. Some runners achieve an ideal physique easily while others need to manipulate their training and dietary programmes to achieve their desired size and shape.

The athlete's power : weight ratio is an important determinant of performance, as all runners are required to move their own body mass (BM) over ground. In sprinting, the emphasis of training is to increase the runner's power with little consideration of the resulting gain in mass. Typically, sprinters have a high lean body mass capable of producing high power outputs over short distances (see Chapter 1). These runners often undertake extensive resistance training programmes designed to increase their muscularity and enhance speed and strength (see Chapter 4). Like many athletes involved in regular strength training programmes, sprinters often focus their dietary interests on protein intake and special supplements that claim to enhance the gain of lean body mass. However, carbohydrate is the major macronutrient needed to fuel intense training sessions

and recovery. As discussed below, protein requirements are easily met by the high-energy intakes that
are typical of runners undertaking heavy training.
Genetic predisposition, a suitable resistance training
programme and adequate total energy intake are the
factors underlying successful gain of lean body mass.

For long distance runners, body mass becomes the
most important consideration in the power : weight
equation. A small body size reduces the energy cost of
running and may also confer some thermoregulatory
advantages in terms of efficient dissipation of heat
generated by the working muscles. Perhaps more
important, a low level of body fat enhances a runner's
power : weight ratio by minimizing the amount of
'dead (fat) weight' that must be transported. Distance
runners are typically lightly muscled, especially in
the upper body, but are most noted for low levels
of subcutaneous fat (see Chapter 2) (Fig. 5.1). Many
distance runners strive to achieve minimum body fat
levels, or at least reduce their body fat content below
their 'natural' or 'healthy' level.

Although weight loss efforts often produce a short-
term boost to running physics, this gain must be
balanced against the disadvantages of very low levels
of body fat and the methods used to achieve these.
Excessive training, chronic low energy and nutrient
intake, and psychological distress are often involved
in fat loss strategies. There is evidence that most
female distance runners maintain a constant struggle
to reduce body fat levels and report energy intakes
that are unexpectedly low for their training schedules
(Barr 1987). Furthermore, disordered eating and
impaired body image among female runners are well
documented (Wilmore 1991). Recently the 'female
athlete triad' (the coexistence of disordered eating,
disturbed menstrual function and suboptimal bone
density) has received considerable attention (Yeager
et al. 1993). It appears that female distance runners are
at increased risk of developing one or more of these
problems, and that the causes and outcomes are often
closely linked. Individually or in combination, these
problems can directly impair running performance.
They will also significantly reduce the runner's career
span by increasing their risk of illness and injury,
including bone injuries such as stress fractures (see
Chapter 6). Long-term problems, such as an increased
risk of osteoporosis in later life, and chronic inadequate nutritional status might also be expected.

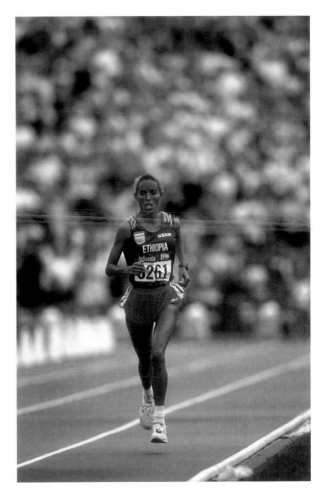

Fig. 5.1 Distance runners are typically lightly muscled,
especially in the upper body, and are most noted for low
levels of subcutaneous fat. Fatuma Roba (Ethiopia) women's
Olympic marathon gold medal winner, Atlanta 1996.
Photo © Allsport.

Runners in all events should be encouraged to set
realistic weight and body fat goals. These are specific
to each athlete and must be judged by trial and error
over a reasonable period of time. Ideal weight and
body fat targets should be set in terms of ranges, and
should consider measures of long-term health and
performance, rather than focusing exclusively on
short-term benefits. In addition, runners should be
able to achieve their targets while eating a diet that is
adequate in energy and nutrients and free of unreason-
able food-related stress. Some racial groups or individuals naturally carry very low levels of body fat,

or can achieve these without paying a substantial penalty. Furthermore, some runners vary their body fat levels over a season so that the lowest levels are achieved only for a specific and short period of time (the competition phase). In general, however, runners should not undertake strategies to minimize body fat levels unless the absence of unacceptable side effects can be demonstrated. Most importantly, the low body fat levels of elite runners should not be considered natural or necessary for recreational and subelite runners. Expert advice from sports medicine professionals, including dietitians, psychologists and physicians, is important in the early detection and management of problems.

Energy and nutrient requirements

The energy requirements of runners vary markedly and are influenced by their body size, the need to lose or gain weight, their phase of growth and development, and training load. The training programmes of runners vary according to event distance, level of competition and the time of the athletic season (see Chapter 4). The results of dietary surveys show that male runners typically report energy intakes varying from 12 to 16 MJ·day^{-1} over prolonged periods (for review see Hawley *et al.* 1995a). The expected energy requirements of female runners should be 20–30% lower than their male counterparts, principally to take into account their smaller size. However, surveys of female runners often report an energy imbalance in which reported intakes of 6–9 MJ·day^{-1} are much lower than expected; sometimes the diets do not seem to cover the costs of the training programme itself (Barr 1987). There appears to be no physiological reason underlying this observation. Rather, it is suspected that concerns about body fat levels cause systematic underreporting of food intake or restricted eating during the period of the food recording. Problems related to disordered eating and unnaturally low body fat levels have already been discussed. In addition, the most common effect of low total energy intake is to restrict the potential for intake of carbohydrate, protein and micronutrient needs.

Prolonged daily training increases the protein requirements of runners. This results from the small contribution of protein oxidation to the fuel requirements of exercise as well as the extra protein needed to support muscle gain and repair of damaged body tissues. While athletes undertaking recreational or light training activities will meet their protein needs within population protein recommended daily intakes (RDIs), guidelines for increased protein intake for runners in heavy training have been set at 1.2–1.6 g·kg^{-1} BM per day (Lemon 1995). Such increases can be met within the increased energy allowances that usually accompany training. Indeed, most dietary surveys report that runners who eat a typical Western diet report protein intakes within or above these goals (Hawley *et al.* 1995a). Although sprint runners whose training regimens include extensive resistance training may eat large amounts of protein-rich foods or buy expensive protein supplements, this is considered largely unnecessary.

The key factors ensuring an adequate intake of vitamins and minerals are a moderate to high energy intake and a varied diet based on nutritious foods. Dietary surveys of runners show that when these factors are in place, reported intakes of vitamins and minerals are well in excess of RDIs and are likely to meet any increases in micronutrient demand caused by training. Thus, generalized micronutrient supplementation is not justified. Furthermore, scientific studies do not support an improvement in performance with such supplementation except in the case where a pre-existing deficiency was corrected (for review see Williams 1989).

Not all runners, however, eat varied diets of adequate energy intake. Energy restriction, fad diets and disordered eating are the typical causes of reduced micronutrient intake. Poor practical nutrition skills, inadequate finances and an overcommitted lifestyle that limits access to food and causes erratic meal schedules may also restrict food range. The best management is to provide the runner with nutrition education to increase the quality and quantity of their food intake. However, a low-dose broad-range multivitamin/mineral supplement may be useful in a situation where a runner is unwilling or unable to make dietary changes, or for a runner who is travelling to locations with an uncertain food supply and eating schedule.

Minerals are the micronutrients at most risk of inadequate intake in the diets of runners. Inadequate iron status can reduce exercise performance via suboptimal levels of haemoglobin, and perhaps iron-related muscle enzymes. Reductions in the haemoglobin levels of distance runners first alerted sports scientists to the issue of the iron status of athletes. However, more recent research has raised the problem of distinguishing true iron deficiency from alterations in iron status measures that are caused by exercise itself (for review see Deakin 1994; Chapter 6). Low iron status in runners is overdiagnosed from single measures of low haemoglobin and ferritin levels. Problems include the failure to account for the dilution effect of the increase in blood volume that accompanies training, and the setting of ferritin levels for athletes with an unreasonably high safety margin. Haemodilution, often termed 'sports anaemia', does not impair exercise performance.

Nevertheless, some runners are at true risk of becoming iron-deficient, but for the same reason as members of the general community: a lower than desirable intake of bioavailable iron. Iron requirements may be increased in some runners as a result of growth needs or to increase gastrointestinal or haemolytic iron losses. Distance runners are likely to incur the highest levels of such losses. However, the most common risk factor among runners is a low energy and/or low iron diet, with females, 'restricted' eaters, vegetarians and runners eating high carbohydrate/low meat diets being likely targets. The heme form of iron found in red meat, liver and shellfish is better absorbed than organic or non-heme iron found in plant foods such as wholegrain cereal foods, legumes and green leafy vegetables. Runners with low iron status, indicated by serum ferritin concentrations lower than 20 ng·ml^{-1}, should be considered for further assessment and treatment. Present evidence does not support the case that low iron status without anaemia reduces exercise performance. However, many runners with such low iron stores, or a sudden drop in iron status, frequently complain of fatigue and inability to recover after heavy training. Many of these runners respond to strategies that improve iron status or prevent a further decrease in iron stores.

A sports medicine expert should undertake evaluation and management of iron status on an individual basis. Prevention and treatment of iron deficiency may include iron supplementation. However, the management plan should include dietary counselling to increase the intake of bioavailable iron, and appropriate strategies to reduce any unwarranted iron loss. Many runners self-prescribe iron supplements;

indeed, mass supplementation of athletes with iron has been fashionable at various times. However, such practices are to be avoided because they exclude the opportunity for a more holistic eating plan. Dietary guidelines for increasing iron intake should be integrated with the runner's other nutritional goals, such as a need for high carbohydrate intake or reduced energy intake. This is where the expertise of a sports dietitian is most useful.

The recent recognition of low bone density in some female distance runners seems contradictory, as exercise is considered to be one of the major factors attenuating the loss of bone mineral content. However, a serious outcome of menstrual disturbances in female athletes is the high risk of either loss of bone density, or failure to optimize the gaining of peak bone mass that should occur during the 10–15 years after the onset of puberty. Optimal nutrition is important to correct the factors that underpin the menstrual dysfunction, as well as those that contribute to suboptimal bone density. Adequate energy intake and the reversal of disordered eating or inadequate nutrient intake are important. Adequate calcium intake is also important for bone health, and requirements may be increased to 1200 mg·day^{-1} in runners with impaired menstrual function. Nutritional strategies to meet calcium needs must be integrated into the total nutrition goals of the athlete. Where adequate calcium intake cannot be met through dietary means, usually through use of low-fat dairy foods or calcium-enriched soy alternatives, a calcium supplement may be considered. For further review of calcium, amenorrhoea, osteopenia and stress fractures see Burke (1994).

Practising competition nutritional strategies

In this section, practices designed to promote optimal competition performance through consideration of fluid and fuel needs will be discussed. Training sessions provide an important opportunity to try out and fine-tune these strategies. Most runners do not replace fluid and fuel needs during prolonged competitive events in accordance with sports nutrition guidelines. While practical considerations may prevent optimal fluid intake during races, at least some of the problems might be overcome by better practice during training sessions. It is noticeable that few runners routinely consume fluids during training. This may reflect the lack of access to fluids, especially sports drinks, at typical training venues. However, an updated knowledge of the physiological and performance advantages of aggressive fluid and carbohydrate replacement should motivate the runner to make his or her own supplies available. By drinking during training, and experimenting with the use of sports drinks during longer workouts, runners will discover the benefits of these strategies, as well as enhance the performance of each training session. Experimentation with fluid and carbohydrate intake may also help runners to tolerate greater fluid volumes, and assist in learning the skills of 'drinking on the run', thus improving the potential for superior strategies on race days.

Nutritional strategies before and during competition

Chapters 1 and 2 summarized the physiological demands of sprinting and distance running, noting some of the factors that could, potentially, cause fatigue or limit performance in such events. Several of the factors limiting performance relate to the fuel and hydration status of the runner. Strategies that reduce the disturbance to fluid and fuel status caused by exercise can reduce or delay the onset of fatigue, thus enhancing performance. These strategies can be undertaken before, during or after exercise, or in combination. Although the following guidelines are based on an extensive body of research, it should be acknowledged that most laboratory studies are conducted using the more research friendly mode of cycling as the exercise protocol. There is some evidence that running elicits different metabolic and performance responses to dietary interventions compared with cycling (Derman *et al.* 1996). However, our present knowledge is not sufficiently sophisticated to allow the preparation of specific guidelines based on these differences. Rather, the following sports nutrition guidelines have been modified slightly to take into account practical issues related to running events.

Fuelling up before competitive events

One aim of competition preparation is to increase the runner's carbohydrate stores to meet the anticipated fuel needs of the event. In high-intensity sprint and middle distance events, muscle carbohydrate is used at very high rates (see Chapters 1 and 2) and performance will be impaired if races are undertaken with inadequate glycogen stores. In the absence of muscle damage, glycogen stores can be restored to normal resting values within 24–36 h, by a high carbohydrate intake (7–10 g·kg^{-1} BM per day) in conjunction with a reduction in exercise volume and intensity. Such preparation is considered sufficient for running events lasting less than 80–90 min (events up to the half-marathon). Runners who compete in longer races (Fig. 5.2) should maximize their prerace muscle glycogen stores by undertaking an exercise–diet programme known as carbohydrate loading (for review see Hawley *et al.* 1997). This tactic has become almost universally linked with the marathon and ultra-distance events. Carbohydrate loading does not increase running speed *per se*, but rather allows the runner to maintain their optimal running pace for a longer time, resulting in an overall improvement in race performance (see Chapter 2).

The original carbohydrate loading protocol, as described by Scandinavian researchers in the late 1960s, used extremes of diet and exercise to first deplete, and then supercompensate muscle and liver glycogen stores. More recently it was demonstrated that well-trained runners might not need to undertake a severe carbohydrate depletion phase to achieve a subsequent increase in glycogen stores (Sherman *et al.* 1981). Instead, a training taper and a high carbohydrate diet (7–10 g·kg^{-1} BM per day) during the 72 h prior to a race appears to achieve similar increases in muscle glycogen to those reported by the more extreme regimens. Thus, in a practical sense, preparation for a long distance event is simply a matter of extending the period of 'fuelling up'. Interestingly, several studies have reported that runners do not have sufficient practical nutritional knowledge to achieve such carbohydrate intakes and may require dietary counselling.

Some elite marathon runners still include a low carbohydrate/high fat 'depletion' phase prior to their loading strategies, believing that the benefits outweigh the severe fatigue that is experienced during this period. The current interest in 'fat adaptation' to improve fat utilization during prolonged endurance events may reopen scientific interest in this idea (see

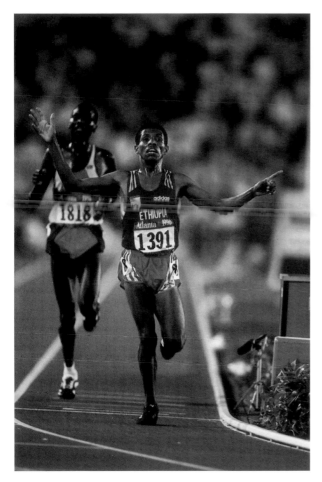

Fig. 5.2 Twenty-four to 36 hours of a high carbohydrate intake and exercise taper is sufficient to fuel up for events up to the half-marathon. Haile Gebrselassie (Ethiopia), men's Olympic 10 000 m gold medal winner, Atlanta 1996 and Paul Tergat (Kenya). Photo © Allsport.

Hawley *et al.* 1998). However, it is too early to provide clear support for any performance benefits following fat adaptation strategies, or to provide guidelines of how they might be utilized by runners. In any case these strategies are likely to be reserved for distance and ultra-distance runners and to be undertaken only for short and well-timed periods.

The pre-event meal offers a last chance to fine-tune fluid and fuel levels prior to a race as well as to ensure gastrointestinal comfort. Runners who have under-taken specific fuelling or loading strategies in the day(s) prior to the event will have achieved optimal muscle carbohydrate stores. Thereafter, should the

event occur early in the day, the major concern is to top-up liver glycogen stores after an overnight fast. Conversely, if training or competition timetables have not allowed optimal recovery from the last exercise session, food eaten in the prerace meal (1–4 h pre-event) may contribute significantly to muscle fuel availability.

The optimal prerace meal varies between runners and is influenced by factors such as the time of day of competition, the need for refuelling and rehydration, food availability and gastrointestinal comfort. The pre-event menu should include carbohydrate-rich low-fat foods, with reduced fibre and protein content being an additional recommendation for runners who experience gastrointestinal discomfort during racing. Fluid intake is also important, especially in preparation for races to be run in hot conditions. While some runners may comfortably consume a larger meal or snack 3–4 h prior to competition, runners involved in early morning events, such as long distance road races, may prefer to consume a smaller snack 1–2 h prior to competition. Liquid meals, such as commercially available supplements, provide a practical alternative for runners who are unable to consume solid foods prior to exercise. Each runner should experiment with various pre-event routines during training to define their optimal strategy. Some suitable prerace meal choices are summarized in Table 5.1.

Fluid and fuel intake during competition

The attenuation of the rise in body temperature during running is an important factor influencing health (see Chapter 6) and performance (see Chapters 1 and 2). Evaporation of sweat from the skin provides a major mechanism to dissipate the heat produced by the working muscle, with a runner's sweat rate being determined by their exercise intensity, state of heat acclimatization and the prevailing environmental conditions. Sweat rates as high as 2–3 l·h⁻¹ have been reported by runners competing in hot and humid conditions. However, in milder environments and with more moderate intensity exercise, typical sweat rates are closer to 1.0–1.2 l·h⁻¹. Unless this fluid is replaced, the runner will eventually become dehydrated. Dehydration is associated with increased thermoregulatory and cardiovascular strain, and an increased perception of effort during exercise.

Table 5.1 Food suggestions for prerace or postexercise recovery. Adapted from Hawley and Burke (1998)

Pre-event meals: high carbohydrate, low fat choices
Breakfast cereal + low-fat milk + fresh/canned fruit
Muffins or crumpets + jam/honey
Pancakes + syrup
Toast + baked beans (note this is a high-fibre choice)
Creamed rice (made with low-fat milk)
Rolls or sandwiches with banana filling
Fruit salad + low-fat fruit yoghurt
Spaghetti with tomato or low-fat sauce
Baked potatoes with low-fat filling
Fruit smoothie (low-fat milk + fruit + yoghurt/ice-cream)
Liquid meal supplement (e.g. Sustagen Sport, Exceed Sports Meal, GatorPro)

Postexercise recovery: 50 g carbohydrate (1–2 portions will provide 1 g·kg⁻¹ BM carbohydrate)
800–1000 ml sports drink
500 ml fruit juice, soft drink or flavoured mineral water
250 ml carbohydrate loader drink
60–70 g packet of jelly beans or jube sweets
3 medium pieces of fruit
3 muesli bars or 2 breakfast bars
1 large Mars bar or chocolate bar (70 g)
3 rice cakes with jam or honey
1 round of jam or honey sandwiches (thick-sliced bread and plenty of jam/honey)
2 crumpets or English muffins with Vegemite/Marmite
Cup of thick vegetable soup with large bread roll
Jaffle/toasted sandwich with banana filling
Some sports bars (check the label)
100 g (1 large or 2 small) American muffin, fruit bun or scones
250 g (1 cup) creamed rice
100 g pancakes (1–2 large) + 30 g syrup

Carbohydrate snacks (50 g) which are also rich in protein (c. 10 g) and other micronutrients
250–350 ml of liquid meal supplement or milk shake/fruit smoothie
Some sports bars (check labels)
2 × 200 g cartons of fruit-flavoured yoghurt
Bowl of breakfast cereal with milk or carton of flavoured yoghurt
250 g tin of baked beans or spaghetti on 2 slices of toast or in jaffle/toasted sandwich
1 round of sandwiches including cheese/meat/chicken in filling, plus 1 piece of fruit
1.5 cups of fruit salad with ½ carton or fruit-flavoured yoghurt or frozen yoghurt
Carton of fruit-flavoured yoghurt or fromage frais and a muesli bar
2 crumpets or English muffins with thick spread of peanut butter
250 g (large) baked potato with cottage cheese or grated cheese filling
150 g thick-crust pizza with lean meat/chicken/seafood and vegetable toppings

The effects of dehydration on exercise performance are most apparent during prolonged exercise in the heat. The detrimental effects of severe levels of dehydration and heat stress have been well publicized through the spectacular collapses of runners, such as Jim Peters in the 1954 Vancouver Empire Games marathon (see Chapter 6) and, more recently, Gabrielle Anderson-Scheiss in the first Olympic marathon for women at the 1984 Los Angeles Games. However, dehydration by as little as 2% of a runner's body mass has been shown to reduce significantly exercise capacity and performance (Walsh *et al.* 1994). The degree of thermoregulatory and exercise impairment appears to be directly related to the fluid deficit, and the runner cannot acquire a tolerance to dehydration as was popularly believed in the past. Dehydration has also been shown to reduce the rate of gastric emptying, which may further compromise exercise performance by decreasing the opportunity for fluid replacement or increasing the risk of gastrointestinal upset. For these reasons, the runner should aim to minimize net fluid losses during all training and competition sessions, particularly by considering the opportunity to consume fluid during sessions lasting longer than 30–40 min.

History has seen considerable changes to the guidelines and practice of fluid intake during running. Early advice to runners ranged from extreme avoidance of drinking to the intake of small fluid volumes. Such conservatism was ensured by the rules of the International Amateur Athletic Federation (IAAF) that governed intake during distance races (see Fig. 5.3). More recently, the debate has concerned the choice of beverages as well as the terminology of fluid intake guidelines.

In terms of optimal hydration, athletes are advised to consume fluids to keep pace with sweat losses, or at least 80% of total sweat losses. However, in most competition and training situations, runners are limited to drinking what is practical rather than optimal. This appears to be between 300 and 800 ml of fluid per hour in most running events.

Even where drinks are made available to runners at aid stations during a race, several practical factors govern total fluid consumption. As drinking during races occurs literally 'on the run', each runner must balance their intake against the possibility of gastrointestinal discomfort or upset, as well as the time lost in slowing down to approach an aid station and to consume the fluid (Coyle & Montain 1992). Many runners appear to consider that the time lost by slowing down or stopping to drink to be greater than the potential benefits to performance with better hydration. Although the top runners in a race may ultimately take a conservative approach to fluid intake because of tactical needs, better hydration strategies are usually possible and are recommended for the rest of the field. This is especially relevant for recreational runners for whom safety and enjoyment are the key priorities.

Despite prerace tactics to maximize fuel levels, many endurance and ultra-endurance events challenge the runner's carbohydrate stores. Carbohydrate intake during such exercise may benefit performance by preventing hypoglycaemia in those individuals susceptible to small changes in blood glucose concentration, and/or by supplying additional fuel for muscle glucose oxidation. Observations of performance benefits following carbohydrate intake were made as far back as the 1920s, during field studies of the Boston marathon (for review see Hawley *et al.* 1995b). In fact, our current guidelines for carbohydrate intake during endurance events are not new. Over the last 30 years numerous studies have reported benefits to endurance capacity and/or performance in prolonged running events when carbohydrate is consumed (for review see Hargreaves 1999). The most recent studies have suggested that benefits may also be seen in events as short as 1 h, even when a runner's fuel status does not appear to be challenged (Millard-Stafford *et al.* 1997).

Despite the availability of supportive scientific data, it is only in the last decade that opportunities to consume carbohydrate and fluid freely during distance events have become universally recommended or allowed.

Figure 5.3 shows the evolution of the IAAF rules governing fluid intake during distance running events. Until the latter part of the 1970s distance runners were largely prevented from drinking fluids early in an event, or frequently during the remainder of a race. The recommendations promoting carbohydrate intake have only been included in official IAAF rules since 1990. Guidelines from key sports science organizations, such as the American College of Sports Medicine (ACSM 1985, 1987) have shown a similar evolution. The initial focus of these guidelines was

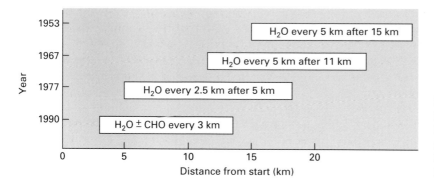

Fig. 5.3 The evolution of the International Amateur Athletic Federation rules governing the intake of fluids during long distance running. Reproduced with permission from Hawley *et al.* (1995b).

to maximize fluid replacement during distance running events and protect against any impairment of gastric emptying that might occur when solutes are added to a drink. Although early studies showed that, compared to plain water, the ingestion of mildly concentrated (2.5% carbohydrate) drinks impaired gastric emptying, there are now many reports that carbohydrate drinks of 4–8% concentration are emptied rapidly and do not compromise fluid replacement.

Commercial sports drinks are manufactured using a combination of carbohydrate types (glucose, sucrose, glucose polymers, etc.) to achieve a palatable beverage with a carbohydrate content within this range, and a moderate (10–25 mmol·l⁻¹) sodium concentration. These sports drinks provide a practical way to achieve carbohydrate and fluid needs during exercise and postexercise recovery. The most recent ACSM guidelines (ACSM 1996) promote the use of such drinks during races, particularly those lasting longer than 1 h. Although earlier guidelines promoted generic fluid intake schedules for runners, it is now recognized that runners should experiment to find a strategy and fluid intake opportunities that suit their own needs. Race organizers, coaches and trainers should assist in making fluids available during events or training sessions.

It should be recognized that gastrointestinal discomfort or upset is a problem in many sports, particularly running. Gastrointestinal problems that occur during exercise involve both the upper and lower intestinal tracts. In addition to the mode of exercise, factors that have been identified as increasing the risk or severity of gastrointestinal problems include being female, undertaking exercise at high intensities (i.e. race pace), being undertrained or dehydrated, and

consuming certain foods or fluids before or during exercise. Runners who experience such problems may be able to adjust their diets, training status or running pace to seek relief. In some cases, medical management may be required.

Recovery after training and competition

In most track events, ranging from sprint to 10 000 m races, competition is conducted as a series of heats and finals. Depending on the level of competition, a runner may be required to compete in a number of events over a day or days (e.g. the Olympic Games). Even where runners compete in a weekly competition (e.g. cross country season or the IAAF Grand Prix series), optimal recovery is desired to allow the runner to undertake training between races. Outside the competitive season, the training schedules of most serious runners involve multiple daily workouts. The value of achieving rapid recovery between training sessions is clear, and recovery strategies must consider the extent and type of nutritional stresses involved as well as the time interval between sessions.

With regard to fuel stores, the key dietary factor for muscle glycogen resynthesis is the amount of carbohydrate a runner consumes. As glycogen recovery is not maximized until carbohydrate intake occurs, rapid refuelling is promoted by the intake of carbohydrate as soon as is practical after the completion of a training session or race. This maximizes the effective recovery time between workouts and competition and is important when the interval between sessions is less than 8 h. Guidelines for maximum recovery promoted an immediate postexercise intake of at least 1 g carbohydrate·kg⁻¹ BM to begin the refuelling process, and a daily carbohydrate intake target intake of 7–10 g·kg^{-1} BM (for review see Burke 1996). The runner will need to be organized to have carbohydrate-rich snacks or meals available after workouts or races. There is some evidence that carbohydrate sources with a high glycaemic index are better at promoting glycogen storage. However, other factors in choosing recovery meals and snacks include appetite appeal and the ease of preparation or eating. Carbohydrate-rich foods and fluids that contain protein and micronutrients will assist the runner to achieve other nutritional goals. Some suitable postexercise snacks are summarized in Table 5.1. Studies have shown that acute refuelling strategies promote faster recovery and better exercise capacity/performance on a subsequent performance trial.

It is interesting that longitudinal studies of chronic high carbohydrate intake have failed to show clearcut benefits to training adaptation and performance compared with more moderate carbohydrate diets. Generally, the results from these studies have shown that carbohydrate intakes, consistent with the guidelines above, promote better recovery of muscle glycogen levels during periods of heavy training. However, there is no evidence of a consistent and significant enhancement of performance after a very high carbohydrate intake (10 g·kg^{-1}·day^{-1}), nor an impairment of performance, in athletes ingesting a moderate (5 g·kg^{-1}·day^{-1}) carbohydrate diet (for review see Sherman & Wimer 1991). It has been suggested that athletes may adapt to the lower carbohydrate intake and muscle glycogen depletion. However, it is also likely that the protocols used to measure performance in these studies were not sufficiently sensitive to detect the differences between the groups, and that the studies were not conducted over sufficiently long periods to elicit clear differences in performance. The topic is confused by some overlap between what are considered 'moderate' and 'high' carbohydrate intakes.

In any case, there is clear evidence from studies of acute dietary manipulation that endurance and performance are enhanced when body carbohydrate stores are optimized, and that carbohydrate depletion causes an impairment of performance. Furthermore, there is anecdotal evidence, including comments from the chronic training studies, that athletes complain of tiredness and muscle fatigue during periods of

training when their intake of dietary carbohydrate is insufficient. Therefore, the recommendation that runners should consume a high (> 5 g·kg^{-1}·day^{-1}) carbohydrate diet to cover the fuel cost of their training programme and recovery is logical and further long-term studies are awaited to test the benefit of this strategy.

Rehydration is also important in the postexercise recovery because runners will be at least mildly dehydrated at the end of their session. From a practical standpoint, the success of postexercise rehydration is dependent on how much the runner drinks, and then how much of this is retained and re-equilibrated within body fluid compartments. It may take up to 24 h for complete rehydration following fluid losses of 2–5% of body mass. With regard to voluntary fluid intake, flavoured drinks may encourage greater intake than plain water. Urine losses appear to be minimized by the appropriate replacement of lost electrolytes, particularly sodium. The inclusion of sodium in a rehydration drink may be an important strategy in the rapid recovery of moderate to high fluid deficits. However, the optimal sodium level is about 50–80 mmol·l^{-1}, as found in oral rehydration solutions used in the treatment of diarrhoea. This is considerably higher than the concentrations found in commercial sports drinks and may be unpalatable to many runners. The consumption of salty carbohydrate-rich foods, such as bread, breakfast cereals or rice, and pasta meals with added salt, will replace sodium losses; creatively planned meals and snacks may fulfil all postexercise recovery needs simultaneously. As caffeine and alcohol promote diaeresis, consumption of large amounts of alcoholic and caffeine-containing drinks may also impair rapid fluid restoration (for review see Maughan *et al.* 1997).

Nutritional supplements for runners

Surveys suggest that at least 50% of athletes use supplements promoted via health food shops, sports magazines and Internet sites. The ever-growing range of products can be divided into two separate categories: sports supplements and nutritional ergogenic aids (Burke & Heeley 1994). Sports supplements may be considered as products that address the special nutritional needs of athletes. This category includes sports drinks, sports bars, liquid meal supplements

Table 5.2 Dietary supplements used by runners. Adapted from Burke and Heeley (1994)

Supplement	Description	Sports-related use
Sports drink	4–8% carbohydrate drink (mixture of carbohydrate types) 10–25 mmol·l⁻¹ sodium. Palatable taste to encourage fluid intake	1 Optimal delivery of fluid + carbohydrate during training and races 2 Rehydration and refuelling after training and races
High carbohydrate supplement or gel	20–25% carbohydrate drink or 60–70% carbohydrate gel (carbohydrate polymers). Gels presented in convenient tear-open package	1 Supplement to high-carbohydrate diet 2 Carbohydrate loading 3 Refuelling after races and training 4 Carbohydrate intake during prolonged races and training, higher CHO intake
Liquid meal	Drink with high-carbohydrate moderate protein and low-fat content. Usually supplies RDIs of vitamins and minerals in 500–1000 ml	1 High energy/carbohydrate/nutrient supplement 2 Prerace carbohydrate intake 3 Refuelling and recovery after races and training 4 Portable nutrition for travelling runner
Sports bar	Convenient and known serving of carbohydrate, usually with low–moderate fat and protein content. Often supplemented with vitamins and minerals	1 High energy/carbohydrate/nutrient supplement 2 Prerace carbohydrate intake 3 Refuelling and recovery after races and training 4 Portable nutrition for travelling runner
Vitamin/mineral supplement	Broad range, 1–5 × RDI of vitamins and minerals	1 Micronutrient support for restricted energy diet 2 Micronutrient support for restricted variety diets 3 Micronutrient support for unreliable food supply (e.g. travel)
Iron supplement	Large doses of ferrous salts	1 Supervised prevention or treatment of iron deficiency
Calcium supplement	Calcium salt in RDI amounts	1 Calcium supplementation in low-energy or low-dairy food diet 2 Assistance in the treatment or prevention of osteopenia

and micronutrient supplements which are part of a prescribed dietary plan (Table 5.2). Many of these products are specially designed to help a runner meet specific needs for energy and nutrient, including fluid and carbohydrate, in situations where everyday foods are not practical. This is particularly relevant for intake immediately before, during or after exercise. These supplements can be shown to improve performance when they allow a runner to achieve their sports nutrition goals. However, they are more expensive than normal food, a consideration that must be balanced against the convenience they provide.

Nutritional ergogenic aids, products that promise a direct and 'supra-physiological' benefit to sports performance, are the supplements that seem to most fascinate runners. These products continually change in popularity, and include mega-doses of vitamins and some minerals, free-form amino acids, ginseng and other herbal compounds, bee pollen, inosine and carnitine. In general, these supplements have been poorly tested or have failed to live up to their claims when rigorous testing has been undertaken.

Table 5.3 Nutritional ergogenic aids with scientific support for use by runners

Supplement	Dose and mode of action	Supported uses
Caffeine	$5-6$ mg·kg^{-1} taken *c.* 1 h prior to exercise. Caffeine affects numerous body tissues in a variety of ways, causing difficulty in isolating a specific mechanism for any observed changes. Effects include stimulation of central nervous system, increase in epinephrine release and activity, increase in cyclic-AMP activity, increase in lipolysis leading to enhanced fat oxidation and glycogen sparing in first 20 min of prolonged exercise	Studies support performance enhancements in prolonged moderate-intensity events (> 90 min), high-intensity events of *c.* 20 min duration and short very high intensity exercise of *c.* 5 min duration. Studies using specific running events are required. Considerable individual variability in response warrants further research and specific experimentation by runners who intend to use caffeine. High doses of > 9 mg·kg^{-1} may produce urinary caffeine levels which contravene IOC doping laws. Doses of 13 mg·kg^{-1} may cause negative side effects. Observed race practices in endurance events (small doses of caffeine during the last stages of race by consuming cola drinks) merit research. For further information see Graham & Spriet (1991); Spriet (1997)
Bicarbonate	300 mg·kg^{-1} taken $1-2$ h prior to exercise. Increases blood bicarbonate levels and pH. May increase tolerance to production of H$^+$ ions via anaerobic glycolysis by enhancing extracellular buffering capacity. Gastrointestinal upsets are often reported and may be reduced by the intake of large volumes of fluid ($1-2$ l) with the bicarbonate dose	Meta-analysis of bicarbonate studies confirms that bicarbonate supplementation enhances capacity for high-intensity exercise of $2-8$ min (see Matson & Tran 1993). Sports-specific studies are required to confirm use in running races in competitive situations. Events likely to benefit from bicarbonate loading are 800 and 1500 m races; with one study supporting this benefit (Wilkes *et al.* 1983). The effect of repeated doses of bicarbonate need to be studied because most middle distance competitions require heats and semifinals to decide the ultimate winner. Gastrointestinal problems may be increased by multiple loading events. For further information see Horswill (1995)
Creatine	Loading: $20-30$ g in multiple doses (e.g. 4×5 g) for 5 days Maintenance dose: $2-5$ g·day^{-1} Loading dose significantly increases muscle creatine and creatine phosphate levels in *c.* $60-70\%$ of people Weight gain of about 1 kg occurs with loading as a result of fluid retention. Creatine phosphate serves a number of important purposes in exercise metabolism; the most well-known role is the provision of ATP in rapid turnover by the phosphagen power system	Studies show that creatine loading enhances the performance of exercise involving repeated high-intensity workouts with short recovery intervals (< 2 min recovery). Performance benefits are seen only in subjects who experience significant increases in creatine stores following loading. Most studies have been undertaken in the laboratory and are yet to be confirmed with well-trained and elite athletes in sports-specific situations. No benefits to aerobic endurance have been reported. Creatine supplementation is likely to assist interval training sessions and thus enhance training adaptations. It may also enhance the gain of muscle mass and strength by assisting the effectiveness of resistance training. Therefore, the runners most likely to benefit from creatine supplementation are sprinters and middle distance runners. For further information see Greenhaff (1995); Spriet (1997)

Exceptions to this are creatine, caffeine and bicarbonate, each of which may enhance the performance of certain athletes under specific conditions (Table 5.3).

Each of these supplements has a special role and history in running. For example, the results of early studies of caffeine and endurance performance were quickly popularized by articles in running magazines and observations at marathon events. More recently, the success of British sprinter Linford Christie at the 1992 Barcelona Olympic Games, in part attributed to his use of creatine, helped to fuel the initial interest in this supplement.

Runners should seek expert advice about such supplements to ensure that the appropriate conditions of use apply to their sporting situation, and that correct dosage is taken. At best, most purported nutritional ergogenic aids offer a placebo to runners and, at worst, they represent a waste of considerable amounts of money. In most cases, runners would be better rewarded by directing their resources and interest to a more credible area of sports performance, such as better equipment, improved training techniques, advice about nutrition or psychological preparation.

Nutrition for the travelling runner

Travel is an integral part of the lifestyle of modern runners: many travel nationally and internationally to compete, or to train in special facilities or environments, such as altitude training (see Chapter 4) or heat acclimatization. However, travel presents a number of challenges to sound nutritional practices, including reduced access to suitable food while eating in hotels, restaurants or on aeroplanes, reduced supervision by parents or coaches, and disruption to the usual routine caused by travel. Additional problems in some countries include an unusual food supply, problems with food hygiene and a safe water supply. Runners may also find it difficult to identify acute changes in nutritional needs caused by a sudden change in training load or in environmental conditions. Failure to meet these challenges may result in unwanted weight loss or gain, chronic dehydration and inadequate carbohydrate recovery, nutrient deficiencies and gastrointestinal upsets, including traveller's diarrhoea. An organized nutrition plan assists runners to eat well while travelling, thus reducing the risk of these problems and promoting optimal performance at these key times. Strategies include the organization of menus and meals in advance and taking important food supplies on the trip. Care with food hygiene and exclusive use of bottled water supplies may be necessary.

Conclusions

Sports nutrition combines science and practice to assist runners to be healthy, train effectively and compete optimally. Special nutritional needs must be met within a busy daily timetable and in conjunction with other nutritional goals. Special fluid and food intake strategies before, during and after exercise can improve performance and enhance subsequent recovery and a return to training and/or competition.

References

American College of Sports Medicine (1985) Position statement on prevention of heat injuries during distance running. *Medicine and Science in Sports and Exercise* **7**, vii–ix.

American College of Sports Medicine (1987) Position statement on prevention of thermal injuries during distance running. *Medicine and Science in Sports and Exercise* **19**, 529–533.

American College of Sports Medicine (1996) Position stand: exercise and fluid replacement. *Medicine and Science in Sports and Exercise* **28**, i–vii.

Barr, S.I. (1987) Women, nutrition and exercise: a review of athletes' intake and a discussion of energy-balance in active women. *Progress in Food and Nutrition Science* **11**, 307–361.

Burke, L.M. (1994) Sports amenorrhoea, osteopenia, stress fractures and calcium. In: *Clinical Sports Nutrition* (eds L.M. Burke & V. Deakin), pp. 220–226. McGraw-Hill, Sydney.

Burke, L.M. (1996) Nutrition for post-exercise recovery. *Australian Journal of Science and Medicine in Sport* **29**, 3–10.

Burke, L.M. & Heeley, P. (1994) Dietary supplements and nutritional ergogenic aids in sport. In: *Clinical Sports Nutrition* (eds L.M. Burke & V. Deakin), pp. 227–284. McGraw-Hill, Sydney.

Coyle, E.F. & Montain, S.J. (1992) Carbohydrate and fluid ingestion during exercise: are there trade-offs? *Medicine and Science in Sports and Exercise* **24**, 671–678.

Deakin, V. (1994) Iron deficiency in athletes: identification, prevention and dietary treatment. In: *Clinical Sports Nutrition* (eds L.M. Burke & V. Deakin), pp. 174–199. McGraw-Hill, Sydney.

Derman, K.D., Hawley, J.A., Noakes, T.D. & Dennis, S.C. (1996) Fuel kinetics during intense running and cycling when fed carbohydrate. *European Journal of Applied Physiology* **74**, 36–43.

Graham, T.E. & Spriet, L.L. (1991) Performance and metabolic responses to a high caffeine dose during prolonged exercise. *Journal of Applied Physiology* **71**, 2292–2298.

Greenhaff, P.L. (1995) Creatine and its application as an ergogenic aid. *International Journal of Sports Nutrition* **5**, S100–S110.

Hargreaves, M. (1999) Metabolic responses to carbohydrate ingestion: effects on exercise performance. In: *Perspectives in Exercise Science and Sports Medicine*, Vol. 12. (ed. R. Murray), pp. 93–124. Cooper Publishing, Carmel, Indiana.

Hawley, J.A., Brouns, F. & Jeukendrup, A. (1998) Strategies to enhance fat utilisation during exercise. *Sports Medicine* **25**, 241–257.

Hawley, J.A. & Burke, L.M. (1998) *Peak Performance. Training and Nutritional Strategies for Sport.* Allen & Unwin, Sydney.

Hawley, J.A., Dennis, S.C., Lindsay, F.H. & Noakes, T.D. (1995a) Nutritional practices of athletes: are they suboptimal? *Journal of Sports Science* **13**, S63–S74.

Hawley, J.A., Dennis, S.C. & Noakes, T.D. (1995b) Carbohydrate, fluid and electrolyte requirements during prolonged exercise. In: *Sports Nutrition: Minerals and Electrolytes*, (eds C.V. Kies & J.A. Driskoll), pp. 235–265. CRC Press, Boca Raton, Florida.

Hawley, J.A., Schabort, E.J., Noakes, T.D. & Dennis, S.C. (1997) Carbohydrate loading and exercise performance: an update. *Sports Medicine* **24**, 73–81.

Horswill, C.A. (1995) Effects of bicarbonate, citrate, and phosphate loading on performance. *International Journal of Sport Nutrition* **5**, S111–S119.

Lemon, P.W.R. (1995) Do athletes need more dietary protein and amino acids? *International Journal of Sport Nutrition* **5**, S39–S61.

Matson, L.G. & Tran, Z.T. (1993) Effects of sodium bicarbonate ingestion on anaerobic performance: a meta-analytic review. *International Journal of Sport Nutrition* **3**, 2–28.

Maughan, R.J., Leiper, J.P. & Shirreffs, S.M. (1997) Factors influencing the restoration of fluid and electrolyte balance after exercise in the heat. *British Journal of Sports Medicine* **31**, 175–182.

Millard-Stafford, M., Rosskopf, L.B., Snow, T.K. & Hinson, B.T. (1997) Water versus carbohydrate-electrolyte ingestion before and during a 15-km run in the heat. *International Journal of Sport Nutrition* **7**, 26–38.

Sherman, W.M., Costill, D.L., Fink, W.J. & Miller, J.M. (1981) Effect of exercise–diet manipulation on muscle glycogen and its subsequent utilisation during performance. *International Journal of Sports Medicine* **2**, 114–118.

Sherman, W.M. & Wimer, G.S. (1991) Insufficient dietary carbohydrate during training: does it impair performance? *International Journal of Sport Nutrition* **1**, 28–44.

Spriet, L.L. (1997) Ergogenic aids: recent advances and retreats. In: *Perspectives in Exercise Science and Sports Medicine*, Vol. 10. *Optimising Sports Performance*, (eds D.R. Lamb & R. Murray), pp. 185–238. Cooper Publishing, Carmel, Indiana.

Walsh, R.M., Noakes, T.D., Hawley, J.A. & Dennis, S.C. (1994) Impaired high-intensity cycling performance time at low levels of dehydration. *International Journal of Sports Medicine* **15**, 392–398.

Wilkes, D., Gledhill, N. & Smyth, R. (1983) Effect of acute induced metabolic acidosis on 800 m racing time. *Medicine and Science in Sports and Exercise* **15**, 277–280.

Williams, M.H. (1989) Vitamin supplementation and athletic performance: an overview. *International Journal of Vitamin and Nutrition Research* **30**, 161–191.

Wilmore, J.H. (1991) Eating and weight disorders in the female athlete. *International Journal of Sports Nutrition* **1**, 104–117.

Yeager, K.K., Agostini, R., Nattiv, A. & Drinkwater, B. (1993) The female athlete triad: disordered eating, amenorrhea, osteoporosis. *Medicine and Science in Sports and Exercise* **25**, 775–777.

Recommended reading

Hawley, J. & Burke, L. (1998) *Peak Performance: Training and Nutritional Strategies for Sport.* Allen & Unwin, Sydney.

Maughan, R.J. (1994) Physiology and nutrition for middle distance and long distance running. In: *Perspectives in Exercise Science and Sports Medicine*, Vol. 7. *Physiology and Nutrition for Competitive Sport*, (eds D.R. Lamb, H.G. Knuttgen & R. Murray). pp. 329–371. Cooper Publishing Group, Carmel, Indiana.

Maughan, R.J. & Horton, E.S. (eds) (1995) Current issues in nutrition in athletics. *Journal of Sports Science* (special issue), Vol. 13.

Williams, C. & Gandy, G. (1994) Physiology and nutrition for sprinting. In: *Perspectives in Exercise Science and Sports Medicine*, Vol. 7. *Physiology and Nutrition for Competitive Sport*, (eds D.R. Lamb, H.G. Knuttgen & R. Murray). pp. 55–98. Cooper Publishing Group, Carmel, Indiana.

Chapter 6

Medical considerations

for runners

While runners are not immune to the myriad of medical conditions that also afflict sedentary non-athletes, there are some conditions which are specific to exercising populations. In this chapter some of the more common medical problems that runners may develop are considered.

The gastrointestinal system

The most common gastrointestinal problems that affect runners, especially during competition, are increased bowel activity causing mild but irritating diarrhoea, the so-called 'runner's trots', and progressive nausea and a disinclination to either eat or drink, especially during the last third of long distance races.

Runner's 'trots'

Between 20 and 40% of runners report abdominal cramps, diarrhoea or the urge to defecate during or after competitive running, symptoms that occur more frequently in men than in women. The physiological mechanisms that explain why gastrointestinal symptoms develop during running are not known. Exercise *per se* is not the likely cause as these symptoms are more common in runners than in either cyclists or swimmers. It is likely that it is a combination of the increased mechanical mixing caused by the bouncing action of running and the elevated concentrations of some circulating hormones that increase bowel motility. Symptoms are also more common in runners who become severely dehydrated (> 4% of body mass) during competition. However, not all runners develop these symptoms so other predisposing factors may need to be present.

One such factor may be mild milk or other food intolerance. Milk (lactose) intolerance may be present in up to 66% of persons with the irritable bowel syndrome and probably in a large number of runners with the 'trots' who may be cured by avoiding all dairy produce for at least 24 h before competition. It is likely that persons who are milk-intolerant have reduced amounts of the enzyme lactase in the small intestine and are lactose-intolerant. Persons with lactase deficiency develop bloating, flatulence, belching, cramps and a watery explosive diarrhoea when they ingest dairy produce.

Individuals who develop the 'trots' during running should initially stop eating dairy products for up to 48 h before competition. If this then prevents the 'trots', the correct cause has been identified. If not, the possibility that the runner is sensitive to another substance, possibly fructose, must be considered. Another tip is for the runner to eat a low-residue diet for 24–48 h before competition so that the colon is relatively empty when starting a race.

Bloody diarrhoea after exercise

As many as 30% of runners may have bloody stools after competitive running. At present the cause of the bleeding is unknown, as even detailed investigations in some runners have failed to identify a mechanism that would explain the bleeding. There is evidence of bleeding from the colon (haemorrhagic colitis), a condition common in younger faster runners, particularly when they have suddenly increased their training or competitive running. However, it usually resolves within 3 days. The condition has been found in triathletes and cyclists, but does not occur in walkers, and seems to be more frequent in runners who ingest analgesic drugs before or after a race. It is also more frequent in those who run very long distances; up to 85% of ultra-marathon runners develop blood in their stools after racing. The volume of blood lost is, however, inconsequential. Thus, it is unlikely to be an important source of blood loss and could not explain the development of iron deficiency and anaemia in runners.

If haemorrhagic colitis persists beyond 3 days medical advice should be sought. Causes of bloody diarrhoea that will require medical or, possibly, surgical intervention include bowel infections and bowel tumours. If no cause is found the runner should be encouraged to avoid anti-inflammatory drugs for 12–24 h and aspirin for 2–3 days before a particularly heavy training session or competition.

Nausea during or after running

Intense or prolonged running frequently causes mild nausea and a decreased appetite during, and for a few hours after exercise. In some runners vomiting may occur, particularly during or after a hard work-out or race. One study found that 6% of runners complained of nausea or retching after racing, while 50% had a reduced appetite for up to 2 h after hard competition. After an easy run, the proportion of runners who reported an increase, decrease or no change in appetite was about the same. The effects could be caused by gastro-oesophageal reflux of stomach contents induced by the mechanical effects of running. Studies show that intra-abdominal pressures rise substantially during running, perhaps sufficient to promote reflux.

However, another possibility is that some cases of nausea in marathon and ultra-marathon runners may be caused simply by motion sickness resulting from the incessant up-and-down movement of the head for hours on end. In such runners the prescription of antinausea medication (prochlorperazine maleate, e.g. 5 mg Stemetil) taken about 1 h before the athlete expects to become ill and again every 2 h until exercise stops, has been helpful. Some runners may need higher doses. Interestingly, susceptibility to motion sickness increases with increasing levels of fitness.

The haematological system

Iron deficiency in runners

A popular belief among medical practitioners is that long distance runners, females in particular, appear to be especially prone to the development of iron deficiency which may present as an iron-deficiency anaemia. Iron is needed for three major body processes: the formation of haemoglobin, which binds with oxygen thereby carrying the oxygen from the lungs to the muscles; the formation of myoglobin, which stores and transports oxygen in the muscle cells; and for a group of enzymes known as the ferrochromes, which exist in the mitochondria and

whose function is essential for the production of adenosine triphosphate (ATP).

Total body iron stores are about 4.0 g, of which 2.7 g is present in haemoglobin, 1 g is present as ferritin or haemosiderin in the liver and bone marrow, and 0.3 g is found in myoglobin and the mitochondrial enzymes. The first stores to be depleted in iron deficiency are the liver and bone marrow iron stores. Only when those two stores are depleted does the iron content of the mitochondrial ferrochromes start to fall, and only then do blood haemoglobin levels fall. Thus anaemia, diagnosed as a fall in the blood haemoglobin content, is probably the final, not the first, indication of body iron deficiency.

Body iron stores can be assessed either directly, by biopsy of the bone and measurement of its iron content, or they can be estimated by measurement of the levels of ferritin in the bloodstream. At least in untrained individuals, the ferritin levels in the blood bear a direct relationship to the size of the body iron stores and are high when body iron stores are replete, and low when body iron stores are depleted. However, this relationship appears to be altered in runners so that blood ferritin levels may not be an accurate measure of the body iron stores in those who run regularly.

Low blood ferritin concentrations (below 30–50 ng·ml^{-1}) have been reported in as many as 20% of male competitive long distance runners. The incidence of low blood ferritin levels among competitive female runners may be even higher; several studies report that 60–80% of female runners had subnormal blood ferritin levels. Recent studies have confirmed these findings by directly measuring the bone marrow iron stores. Scandinavian and Israeli researchers found the virtual total absence of bone marrow iron stores in different groups of long distance runners, all of whom had normal blood haemoglobin levels. Originally it was considered that the low serum ferritin levels and the absence of bone marrow iron in these runners must indicate that they were seriously iron-deficient, even though they were not anaemic. However, more recent research has found that runners with very low serum ferritin levels and absent bone marrow iron stores nevertheless had a normal rate of production of red blood cells, whose quality was also normal. The explanation is that as a result of red cell destruction in their feet while they run, runners store iron in their livers rather than in the bone marrow, as do more sedentary humans. Thus, the conventional methods used to diagnose iron deficiency in non-runners are not applicable to runners.

Support for the belief that runners with low blood ferritin concentrations are not iron-deficient comes from studies showing that iron therapy does not improve either the exercise performance, the maximal oxygen uptake ($\dot{V}_{O_{2max}}$) values, or the running speed at the blood lactate turnpoint of different groups of runners (Matter *et al.* 1987), or that the induction of iron deficiency by blood withdrawal does not affect maximum exercise tolerance once blood haemoglobin levels are restored with blood transfusion (Celsing *et al.* 1986).

These studies have concluded that iron therapy should be reserved for runners whose blood haemoglobin levels are subnormal. In the absence of established anaemia, shown by low blood haemoglobin levels, low serum ferritin levels in runners can probably be ignored.

Iron deficiency with anaemia

Once true iron deficiency develops, the haemoglobin content of the red blood cells falls and the cells become smaller, less able to carry oxygen and more fragile, with a reduced life expectancy. Persons with iron-deficiency anaemia suffer from a reduced blood oxygen-carrying capacity, which will cause a reduced $\dot{V}_{O_{2max}}$. With appropriate iron therapy, $\dot{V}_{O_{2max}}$ and running performance improves.

The possible causes of iron-deficiency anaemia in runners have not been established. Possibilities include excessive iron losses in sweat or excessive blood losses in the gastrointestinal tract or in urine because of haematuria, haemoglobinuria, or both. Haemoglobinuria may result from accelerated intra-vascular haemolysis. In some female runners excessive menstrual blood losses may contribute to iron deficiency. Another cause may be impaired gastro-intestinal absorption of ingested iron. A deficient dietary intake must also be considered because runners undergoing intensive training tend to eat high-carbohydrate vegetarian-type diets, which usually have low iron contents (see Chapter 5). In addition, some elite runners, women in particular, may severely restrict their dietary energy intakes or may suffer from disordered eating. However, at present the consensus of opinion is that anaemia in athletes is caused by the same mechanisms that cause anaemia in the sedentary population and that there is no such entity as the anaemia of exercise.

Low haemoglobin levels in athletes without proven iron deficiency ('sports anaemia')

An interesting haematological finding in endurance runners is that they may have subnormal blood haemoglobin levels without other evidence of iron deficiency (Fig. 6.1). In competitors at the 1948 Olympic Games, it was noted that the athletes competing in sports requiring 'great endurance' had the lowest haemoglobin levels. In particular, the endurance athletes in the 1968 Dutch and Australian Olympic teams were found to have blood haemoglobin levels that were lower than those of their team coaches and managers. Of interest was that the Australian athletes with the lowest haemoglobin levels subsequently performed the worst in the Games. Essentially the same findings were reported by Clement *et al.* (1977) for the 1976 Canadian Olympic team.

The cause of these low haemoglobin levels, so-called 'sports anaemia', is currently unknown. As none of the earlier studies measured blood ferritin levels or performed bone marrow biopsies to measure body iron stores, it is not known whether this sports anaemia is caused by iron deficiency or simply to dilution as a result of an increased circulating blood volume. The latter would seem more likely. Nevertheless, a low haemoglobin level in a long distance runner should be considered abnormal and requires investigation and treatment. The possible causes of the anaemia are likely to be the same as those for anaemia in the sedentary population. An increase in blood haemoglobin levels in response to iron therapy would indicate that iron deficiency was the cause of the low haemoglobin level.

Anaemia of early season training

Since 1966 it has been known that individuals who start exercising for the first time, or who undergo a period of very intensive training, develop an anaemia

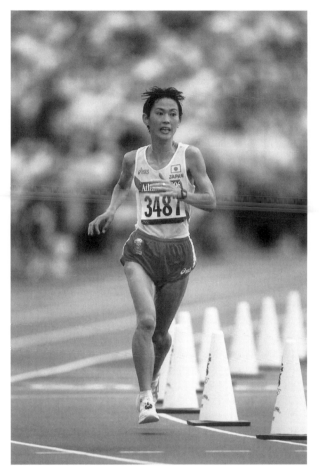

Fig. 6.1 Long distance runners may have subnormal blood haemoglobin levels without other evidence of iron deficiency. Anaemia is more commonly found in female distance runners. Photo © Allsport / M. Hewitt.

which can be quite severe, causing blood haemoglobin levels to fall by up to 18%. This is likely to be caused by an increased rate of red blood cell destruction. The anaemia corrects itself within about 3–8 weeks and can be prevented by eating a high-protein diet (2 g protein·kg^{-1} body mass per day). The anaemia appears to be caused by the release into the bloodstream of a chemical substance, possibly lysolethicin from the spleen, which causes the rapid destruction of a large number of circulating red blood cells. Iron ingestion does not prevent the development of this anaemia. To prevent the anaemia associated with the onset of early season training, runners should increase their dietary protein intakes for the first month or so of training.

Runners and blood donations

A question frequently asked by runners is whether they should donate blood. In donating blood, the runner typically loses three components: 500 ml of fluid; approximately 70 g of haemoglobin (equivalent to 220 mg of iron); and many millions of red blood cells. The fluid loss is rapidly replaced within a matter of hours, but the restoration of red blood cells takes considerably longer: at least 3 weeks and possibly much longer in athletes who are iron-deficient. The runner who does choose to donate blood should probably not exercise on the day of blood donation because of the reduced blood volume, and should avoid hard competition over any distance until his or her haemoglobin level has returned to normal, usually 3–6 weeks after a donation. Runners who wish to donate blood must first have their blood ferritin and haemoglobin levels measured. If the haemoglobin level is normal and the ferritin level is high (> 60 ng·ml^{-1} in a sample collected when the athlete has not run hard for at least 5 days), it is safe to donate blood. Runners should be more careful if blood ferritin levels are low and should take iron supplements and definitely not donate blood if the haemoglobin level is low (< 14 5 g·dl^{-1} in males or 12.5 g·dl^{-1} in females).

The immune system

Exercise and resistance to infection

The risk of infection is increased immediately after competitive racing. In addition, infection is an important feature of the 'overtraining syndrome'. The reasons for this are unknown but probably indicate that the body's immune system, and with it the runner's resistance to infection, is impaired by heavy training and intense competition and by the associated weight loss.

Paradoxically, mild exercise releases a protein, endogenous pyrogen, that causes the body temperature to rise. It is believed that this elevation of body temperature, corresponding to the fever stage of infection, is beneficial because it creates an internal environment that is less favourable for the growth and multiplication of invading bacteria and viruses. In addition, blood levels of the antiviral protein, interferon, increase, as does the activity of 'killer' white cells. Thus, mild exercise should reduce acutely the risk that an athlete develops an infection. A number of studies indeed confirm that moderate exercisers have fewer infections than do non-exercisers (Mackinnon 1998). Surprisingly, chronic training appears not to influence immune function, even in groups of runners who claim to have had fewer infections since they started running. However, much is still to be learned of the influence of exercise and overtraining on the immune system.

Exercise-induced anaphylaxis

There are a small group of runners, and other sportspersons, who develop the life-threatening exercise-associated syndrome of anaphylaxis (Scheffer & Austen 1980; Siegel 1980). Interestingly, the condition may have a familial basis. The syndrome is characterized by the onset during exercise of severe redness, blistering (urticaria) and itchiness of the skin, face, palms and soles, associated with (in decreasing order of frequency) cardiovascular collapse, upper respiratory tract airway obstruction as a result of marked swelling of the throat causing choking and wheezing, and gastrointestinal symptoms including colic, nausea or diarrhoea. There may also be headaches and vertigo, which can persist for up to 3 days after an attack. The attacks, which can last anything from 1 to 4 h, are totally unpredictable. They do not occur with every exercise session and have been reported as frequently as once a month and as infrequently as once every decade. It seems likely that the syndrome occurs in allergic persons only when exercise follows the exposure of that person to a specific protein (antigen) to which he or she is allergic. Antigens that have been identified include shellfish, caffeine and aspirin, wheat, grain flour, celery and even running shoes.

Treatment, which must be given immediately if there is shock or serious respiratory obstruction, must include the subcutaneous injection of adrenaline (epinephrine) and the intravenous injection of antihistamine drugs. The long-term prevention of the condition requires the identification of the specific antigen that provokes the attacks.

Special medical problems in the runner

Dehydration

Perhaps the single most important change in long distance running in the past 50 years has been the realization that fluid and energy must be ingested if competitive performance is to be enhanced and the risk of harm is to be minimized. Thus, prior to 1967, athletes were encouraged *not* to drink, especially during prolonged exercise (see Chapter 5). Fluid ingestion was considered a likely cause of the 'stitch' and was believed to impair performance. In 1955 the then world-record holder in the marathon wrote: 'in the marathon race there is no need to take any solid food at all and every effort should also be made to do without liquid, as the moment food or drink is taken, the body has to start dealing with its digestion, and in so doing some discomfort will almost invariably be felt' (Peters 1955).

Research in the 1970s began to establish that fluid and energy replacement aids performance during exercise and may, perhaps, reduce the risk of certain medical complications during prolonged exercise. As a result of the impact of some of these investigations, most of the popular marathon races around the world now provide fluid at regular intervals during races. In some events, including the 90-km Comrades Marathon in South Africa and the big city marathons in the USA, fluid may be available as frequently as every 2 km for the entire distance of the race.

It would seem probable that this change in the conduct of these races must have impacted on and, in particular, reduced substantially the probability that athletes competing in these events would become dehydrated. In contrast, it would seem almost inconceivable that athletes competing under those conditions could develop significant dehydration. Indeed, it would seem possible that some might drink too much and become *overhydrated* as a result of this major change in fluid provision during exercise.

Despite this change, it continues to be the accepted dogma that severe dehydration is an inevitable consequence of racing in marathons or longer distance races. However, this premise is not well supported by the published evidence; levels of dehydration are modest in most marathon runners and become even lower in runners participating in ultra-marathons, some of whom actually gain weight during these races (for review see Noakes 1993). Thus, rates of fluid ingestion are probably acceptable in most runners, with the increasing probability that the fluid intakes of runners competing in very long races will be *greater* than required.

It would seem that the only runners whose fluid intakes may be inadequate are those who run the fastest in races of between 10 and 42 km. These runners compete at an intensity of 85% of $\dot{V}O_{2max}$, or higher. At these high exercise intensities, rates of gastric emptying and possibly intestinal absorption are likely to be impaired. In addition, high rates of ventilation make the actual process of drinking both difficult and uncomfortable. High pressures inside the abdomen induced by running faster compound this discomfort. The fast running speeds of these elite athletes ensure high metabolic rates and therefore also high sweat rates. It is precisely these runners who require the highest rates of fluid intake during exercise, who also have the greatest difficulty in replacing their fluid losses during exercise.

High running speeds, and the associated high rates of heat production, also cause body temperature to be elevated. When environmental conditions are so severe that they are unable to lose heat at rates equal to their high rates of heat production, these runners risk developing heat-stroke. In contrast, when slower runners, whose rates of both heat production and sweat production are substantially less, are encouraged to drink at high rates during marathon and ultra-marathon races, they risk the development of water intoxication (hyponatraemia).

Fluid overload

Slower runners, especially during ultra-marathon races, have less difficulty in drinking adequately and some may ingest so much that their lives are at risk. For example, by consuming 1000 ml·h^{-1} instead of 500 ml·h^{-1} during an ultra-marathon, some runners have developed the potentially fatal condition known as overhydration, water intoxication or hyponatraemia (low blood sodium concentration) (Noakes 1992). Hyponatraemia was first reported in four athletes competing in ultra-marathons or ultra-triathlons. Of 17 runners who were hospitalized after the 1985 Comrades Marathon (90 km), nine had

hyponatraemia; after the 1987 race 24 such cases were reported. Among these were runners who were critically ill; three nearly died. All these runners were uniquely predisposed to developing the condition because they were unable to excrete the excess fluid they ingested during the exercise bout.

Typically, runners who are affected are not elite competitive runners but those who are completing these ultra-marathons in between 9 and 11 h. Their slow running speeds allow them ample time to drink fluid from the vast number of feeding stations available during these races. But, more importantly, their slow running speeds and resultant low metabolic rates cause them to sweat at much slower rates than those calculated by previous workers, who studied only elite marathon runners. It is clear that sweat rate calculations based on elite runners are erroneous if applied to the average runner of the same body mass, who runs much more slowly. For example, researchers originally believed that if a 50-kg runner loses 5.5 l of sweat during an ultra-marathon taking 5–6 h, then that runner should obviously drink 1 l of fluid every hour to maintain fluid balance. Such a calculation ignores the water lost from glycogen, which may not have to be replaced. Thus the general, but incorrect, rule was devised that a 50-kg athlete should drink 1 l of fluid for every hour of running, and that those who are heavier should drink a little more. We now know that this advice is safe only if the runner is able to finish the race in 5–6 h. A less competitive 50-kg runner who followed that advice but took 10 h to complete the race would finish the race with a fluid credit of about 4 l, enough to cause water intoxication *if the runner is predisposed to the condition.* The finding that the incidence of hyponatraemia is on the increase among slower ultra-marathon runners and triathletes suggests that this is happening more frequently.

In conclusion, while runners and triathletes must be encouraged to drink adequately during exercise, this must be tempered with advice of exactly what is 'adequate'. An adequate fluid intake is one where the sweat and urine losses incurred during exercise are replaced as they occur. Runners need to understand that fluid ingested in excess of losses can be extremely dangerous, potentially much more dangerous than drinking less than required. Water intoxication also impairs performance.

Hyperthermia

The history of the marathon, more than any other sport, is etched with the tragedy of heat-related deaths. The hero of the 1908 Olympics in London, the diminutive Italian, Dorando Pietri, lay in a semicoma desperately close to death for the 2 days following his collapse in the final metres of the marathon. In the 1912 Olympic Games in Stockholm, the Portuguese runner, Lazaro, collapsed from heat-stroke after running 30.58 km (19 miles) and died the next day. Jim Peters, the first marathon runner to break the 2 h 20 min barrier, entered the Vancouver Stadium 15 min ahead of his nearest rival in the 1954 Empire Games marathon, only to collapse before reaching the finishing line. Worse, in accordance with the rules of the day, there were few seconding stations. Those that did exist were unattended, as the officials had chosen to return to the stadium to watch the Landy–Bannister 'Mile of the Century' run 20 min before Peters was due to arrive in the stadium. Since these disasters, there have been three major changes that have reduced the risk of heat-stroke occurring during races.

First, most races are no longer held in the heat of the day as was the case in the 1954 Empire Games marathon. Rather, these races are usually scheduled —with the notable exception of the men's 1984 Olympic marathon—in the early morning or late evening. Secondly, the facilities for providing the athletes with fluid replacement during races have greatly improved. Whereas in the early 1970s, drinking was allowed only after the first 10 km and then only every 5 km, today refreshment (seconding) stations are provided every 2–3 km and often more frequently at the most popular races. Thirdly, runners have become aware of the need to pre-acclimatize by training in the heat if they are to run hot-weather marathons, and of the need to run conservatively in the heat. Despite these measures, however, a small number of runners continue to suffer from heat injury during racing, so that it is important to recognize the condition in order to know how it should be treated and prevented.

Symptoms and diagnosis of heat-stroke

When, during exercise, the previously healthy runner shows evidence of marked changes in mental functioning—for example, collapse with unconscious-ness, a reduced level of consciousness (stupor, coma) or mental stimulation (irritability, aggression, convulsions), in association with a rectal temperature over 41 °C (Peters' was reportedly 42 °C)—the diagnosis is heat-stroke. During the first 48 h after collapse, a rise in blood levels of certain enzymes that leak from the muscles into the blood as a result of heat damage confirms the diagnosis.

The only conditions with which the heat-stroke may initially be confused are heart attack (cardiac arrest), a severe fall in blood glucose levels (hypoglycaemia) or hyponatraemia (water intoxication). In runners with cardiac arrest, the heart has stopped beating and the athlete does not breathe: thus a pulse will not be felt and the chest wall will not move. In contrast, in heat-stroke, the pulse rate is rapid (usually more than 100 beats·min^{-1}), and breathing is more rapid and obvious. Thus, simply feeling the pulse will differentiate between heat-stroke and cardiac arrest.

Identifying hypoglycaemia or hyponatraemia is far more difficult. Indeed, the distinction can be made only on the basis of the rectal temperature, which is usually lower than 40 °C in hypoglycaemia and hyponatraemia, and by measurement of the prevailing blood glucose and sodium concentrations. A simple but practical approach is first to correct any hypoglycaemia in a collapsed runner by giving adequate amounts of glucose intravenously. The athlete with pure hypoglycaemia will recover rapidly with this treatment; the condition of runners with heat-stroke or water intoxication (hyponatraemia) will be unaffected. In practice, the diagnosis of hyponatraemia is usually made on the basis of exclusion; if an athlete is unconscious or severely confused and the rectal temperature is not elevated, the most likely diagnosis is hyponatraemia, especially when the blood glucose concentration is also found to be normal. The diagnosis of hyponatraemia is confirmed by measuring the blood sodium concentration which is usually below 125 mmol·l^{-1} in those runners unconscious as a result of hyponatraemia.

Factors that predispose to heat-stroke are those that disturb the equilibrium between the rate of heat production and that of heat loss. The air temperature, its humidity and the rate of wind movement control the rate of heat loss across the athlete's body. The athlete's body mass and running speed determine the rate of heat production. Thus, the rate of heat production and the risk of heat-stroke is greatest in short distance races, not in the marathon as is commonly believed. Indeed, this is a critical point that is not appreciated by many runners or race organizers. The major factors causing heat-stroke during races are the environmental conditions, the speed at which the athletes run and individual susceptibility. If longer distance races are held when either the wet bulb globe temperature index or the dry bulb temperature is > 23 °C, heat injury will occur to a significant number of competitors regardless of how much they drink and sponge during the race or how they are dressed. Adequate fluid replacement during racing is only one of many factors that reduce risk of heat injury; it is certainly not the only factor and may not even be a very important one.

Other factors that determine the rate at which the athlete loses heat are: clothing, because the more clothing one wears, the less heat one will lose by convection and sweating; the state of heat-acclimatization, because heat-acclimatization increases both the ability to lose heat by sweating and the resistance to an elevated body temperature; and the runner's state of hydration, because dehydration impairs the ability to lose heat by sweating. Finally, it is clear that only certain runners are prone to heat-stroke, for reasons that are at present unknown. It seems likely that they could have a hereditary abnormality of muscle cell metabolism.

The first priority in the treatment of heat-stroke is to lower the body (core) temperature to below 38 °C as quickly as possible because the amount of tissue damage caused by the high body temperature is related to the time during which body temperature exceeds that value. The most effective cooling method is to place the athlete's torso in an ice-cold bath with arms and legs hanging over the sides. This technique induces a rapid fall in temperature of between 1 and 2 °C every 5 min depending on the runner's body composition: small, thin ectomorphic runners with little muscle bulk or body fat content are likely to cool very rapidly, whereas muscular more obese runners are likely to cool more slowly.

As soon as a cooling procedure has been instituted, correction of any dehydration, which is likely to be mild, and possible hypoglycaemia with intravenous fluids and glucose must be considered. Once the rectal temperature has been reduced to below 38.5 °C, active cooling should cease as the change in the rectal

temperature lags behind the core body temperature by 1–2 °C. Persistent cooling below a core temperature of 37 °C is potentially dangerous.

Once the rectal temperature is at or below 38.5 °C, it must be decided whether the athlete needs to be transported to hospital for further cooling and observation in case any of the serious complications of heat-stroke, in particular kidney failure and organ damage, should occur. Most runners will not require this and can be adequately managed in the medical tent at the race finish. Athletes who rapidly regain consciousness with adequate cooling will not be likely to require hospital admission. However, if a runner is sent to hospital, it is important that the body temperature be monitored continuously during transport to hospital and after admission as it tends to rise once the active cooling procedures cease. Finally, runners who develop heat-stroke during exercise need to be counselled regarding the factors that might have contributed to the condition.

Hypothermia

Although many marathons in the Southern hemisphere and in equatorial countries are run in relatively warm to very hot conditions, many in the Northern hemisphere are run in cold conditions. Athletes in these countries need to understand how their bodies regulate temperature when running in the cold. Once body temperature falls below 35 °C, mental functioning is impaired and the blood pressure falls. At temperatures below 33 °C, mental confusion develops and the limb muscles become rigid and immobile. Unconsciousness develops shortly thereafter, leading to death from hypothermia if the body is not rapidly rewarmed.

In reality, only under certain well-defined conditions does the rate of heat loss from the body exceed its rate of production during exercise, thereby leading to hypothermia. Survival in severe environmental conditions is, however, critically dependent on the choice of appropriate clothing as, despite its ability to produce a vast amount of heat during exercise, the body has a relatively limited ability to reduce its rate of energy transfer to the environment. The avoidance of hypothermia when exposed to the cold depends on three important factors: the choice of appropriate clothing; staying dry; and maintaining a high rate of heat production, as occurs during exercise. By way of example, the insulating qualities of different clothes are rated in clothing (CLO) units. Whereas a resting human would need to wear 12 CLO units of clothing to maintain body temperature at −50 °C, when running at 16 km h⁻¹ at the same temperature the same person would be adequately protected by only 1.25 CLO units of clothing. This is little more than normal business attire. Allowance must also be made for clothing that becomes wet, because the insulating properties of clothes are greatly reduced. Unlike air, water is a very poor insulator; that is, it is a very good conductor of heat. This explains why exposure to cold water (less than 10 °C) can induce critical hypothermia in under 30 min in lean swimmers, whereas exposure to still air at the same temperature would induce a feeling of discomfort and coldness but not death.

Alternatively, clothing may become wet, so losing its insulating properties. In reality, hypothermia usually develops as a consequence of all these mechanisms acting in fatal concert. Maintenance of body temperature during exercise in the cold therefore depends on choosing clothing that is appropriate for the predicted rate of energy expenditure in the expected environmental conditions, and keeping the clothing dry, especially if there is a strong wind blowing.

Additional points to remember are that the runner should try to wear sufficient clothing to keep warm, but not so much that they start to sweat profusely, as sweat wets clothing thereby reducing its insulating properties. The runner should also always start running into the wind when fresh so that the wind comes from behind when he or she is tired. In this way the cooling effect of the environment is greatest when the athlete is freshest, running the fastest and therefore generating the most body heat, and least when the athlete is tired, running the slowest and producing the least heat. Always plan to run in well-populated areas so that help is close at hand should hypothermia develop, and never run far enough to become tired enough to have to walk; walking dramatically increases the amount of clothing that must be worn to keep warm at low effective air temperatures. Finally, runners should wear clothing, such as a lightweight rain jacket with a zip-up front and a hood, that is easily adaptable and can be worn either zipped or unzipped and with or without the hood; it should be able to be carried with equal ease. It is also sensible to choose running routes which provide as much shelter from the wind as possible.

So much attention has been paid to the dangers of heat-stroke developing during marathon running that it has only slowly been appreciated that the opposite condition, hypothermia, can also develop in runners. The first documented case of hypothermia in a marathon runner was that of Ledingham *et al.* (1982), who reported a rectal temperature of 34.3 °C in a runner who collapsed in the Glasgow Marathon, which was run under dry but cold conditions (dry bulb temperature 12 °C) with a strong wind of 16−40 km·h⁻¹. Subsequently, Maughan (1985) measured the rectal temperature of 59 runners completing the 1982 Aberdeen Marathon, run under more favourable weather conditions (dry bulb temperature 12 °C; dry with humidity of 75% and a wind speed of about 26 km·h⁻¹). Despite the relatively mild conditions of the race, including the absence of rain, four runners finished the race with rectal temperatures below the normal 37 °C.

There are three factors that predispose an athlete to the development of hypothermia during distance running: the environmental conditions; the athlete's clothing and body build; and the speed at which he or she runs. Calculations indicate that the effective air temperatures prevailing in the three marathon races described above, in which runners became hypothermic, would have been between 1 and 3 °C. Were those conditions to prevail for the duration of the race, runners running at 16 km·h⁻¹ would need to wear clothing providing about 1.1 CLO units, whereas those who were reduced to a walk (5 km·h⁻¹) during the run would require approximately 2 CLO units of insulation. This is approximately twice the insulating properties (warmth) of normal business attire. In reality it is probable that most runners are unaware of the dangers of marathon running in the cold so that they fail to wear clothing that provides sufficient insulation, particularly under conditions of wet, cold and especially wind.

Runners who have little body fat and are not muscular will likely be most affected by the cold, and the most likely to become hypothermic. The thin ectomorphic African runners who currently dominate world athletics also complain of difficulty when running in cold conditions.

The role of running speed in protecting against hypothermia has already been discussed. The important practical point is that the change from running to walking has a marked effect on the clothing needed to maintain body temperature even at relatively mild effective temperatures. Thus, clothing with at least four times as much insulation is required to maintain body temperature at rest at an effective air temperature of 0 °C as when running at 16 km·h⁻¹. For this reason it is most probable that hypothermia will occur in those marathon runners who are lean, lightly muscled and lightly clothed and who become fatigued and are forced to walk for prolonged periods during marathon races run in effective air temperatures of less than 5 °C. Prevention of the condition is simply to ensure that extra clothing is available should the athlete be forced to walk when racing in cold conditions. Similarly, rain suits should be worn whenever an athlete begins to walk in the rain.

Common running injuries

The common running injuries discussed in this chapter are those that occur to bone, tendon and muscle. Additional information about other injuries can be found in the list of recommended reading.

Bone injuries

Stress fractures

Unlike the common bone fractures occurring in contact sports, such as American football and rugby, in which a single external blow causes the bone to fracture, the runner's bone may fracture as a result of repetitive minor trauma accumulating over weeks or months. These injuries occur in runners whose bones are too weak (for reasons detailed below) to cope with the load to which they are exposed in running.

The tibia (large shin bone) appears to be the most vulnerable to stress fractures. The tibia is followed, in order of frequency of occurrence, by the metatarsals (toe bones), the fibula (small calf bone), the femur (thigh bone), the navicular (ankle bone) and the pubic bone (groin).

The pain associated with a stress fracture is usually bearable when at rest or when walking but as soon as

any running is attempted it becomes quite unbearable and running is impossible. This is the single most important factor in establishing the diagnosis.

The diagnosis of a stress fracture is quite simple.
• The injury is usually of quite sudden onset and there is no history of external violence. An injury that prevents running is almost always a stress fracture.
• The runner will find that standing on one leg may be painful, if not impossible (fracture of the pelvis). Alternatively, hopping on the injured leg is almost always painful in the other fractures. The site of pain corresponds to the site of the fracture.
• Extreme tenderness, localized to the bone, is felt when the injured site is pressed with the fingertips.
• The injury heals itself completely within 3 months of complete rest.

A general rule for the rate of healing is that the further the site is from the centre of gravity of the body, the shorter the healing period. Thus, stress fractures of the foot can heal within 5 weeks, whereas those of the pelvis can take up to 5 months before recovery is complete. Few runners will accept a lengthy rest period without some visible evidence that the diagnosis is correct so it is usual for X-rays and bone scans to be performed. Both, however, are not without their own drawbacks. X-rays will often fail to reveal the presence of a stress fracture if they are taken earlier than 3 weeks after the initial injury. In effect, the fracture is too small to be imaged. Only with the formation of new bone, which is more dense than the old bone it replaces, does the fracture show as a dense line on the X-ray.

If a stress fracture is suspected, bone scanning is only necessary either if the injury fails to heal within 5 weeks for smaller bones to 12 weeks for larger bones, such as the femur, tibia and pelvis, or if it recurs within a few weeks of the runner starting to run again. Neither of these are features of a conventional stress fracture and would indicate the need for a thorough evaluation to exclude another cause of pain, such as bone cancer, unrelated to running.

The exact reason why stress fractures occur is not known, but there appears to be an abnormal concentration of stress at a particular site in the bone which is insufficiently strong at that site to resist those forces. The initial response in bones subjected to increased loading is the activation of specialized cells, osteoclasts, whose function it is to cause bone resorption.

During this process bone minerals are reabsorbed by the body. This is known as osteoclonal excavation. During this phase bone strength is likely to be reduced, placing the bone at increased risk of fracture.

This process of bone resorption passes gradually into a phase in which new bone is laid down by other specialized bone cells, the osteoblasts. Stress fractures and bone strain develop in those whose bones either undergo excessive osteoclonal excavation or whose osteoblastic response is either delayed or initially ineffectual. There are various risk factors that are associated with the incidence of stress fractures.

Women are more prone to stress fractures than men. It has been shown that the frequency of stress fractures in women is up to 12 times higher than in men and women who experience menstrual abnormalities are especially at risk. Most stress fractures occur in novice runners, or in competitive runners who suddenly increase their training load, run one or more very long races, return too quickly to heavy training or sustain a very heavy training and racing programme for many months. Hard training during the early period of bone weakening is more likely to cause a fracture. Novice runners are particularly vulnerable 8–12 weeks after training begins, for it is then that their increased muscle and heart fitness allows them to train much harder at the exact time when their bones are not yet strong enough to cope with the added stress of heavier training. Another adverse feature of suddenly increasing the training distance is that it causes accumulated muscle fatigue which may then reduce the muscles' ability to absorb fatigue which may reduce the muscles' ability to absorb shock—a function which is then passed on to the bones, which are thus more likely to fracture.

Excessively hard running shoes, in particular training spikes in track athletes or shoes with compacted ethylene vinyl acetate, may be a factor explaining this injury. However, it seems that shoes have less of a role in this injury than do major errors in training methods.

Three principal genetic factors are associated with stress fractures: the high-arched foot which fails to absorb shock adequately and is associated with fractures of the femur (thigh bone) and metatarsals (toe bones); the pronating low-arched foot which causes abnormal biomechanical function in the lower limb, predisposing the tibia (large calf bone) and the

fibula (small calf bone) to fractures; and leg-length inequalities.

There is growing evidence that the bones of most female athletes who have abnormal menstrual patterns are likely to become weaker. This happens first because the blood levels of the female hormone, oestrogen, which is required for normal bone mineralization, are depressed and, secondly, because their dietary calcium intake may be too low to maintain normal bone mineral content. Their weaker bones are more prone to bone strain injuries and stress fractures. Studies have shown that the dietary calcium intakes of athletes with shin soreness (stress fractures or tibial or fibular bone strain) are abnormally low and could be a predisposing factor for the injury. Alternatively, it may be that the diets of these injured runners are inadequate in many dietary components (energy, protein and minerals), not only calcium (see Chapter 5).

The only treatment required for most stress fractures is 6–12 weeks' rest. Because these fractures seldom become unstable and are therefore not liable to go out of alignment, they do not need to be placed in plaster of Paris. Some form of bandaging may reduce discomfort in the early weeks following injury. There is one exception to the general rule that stress fractures do not need to be immobilized. A stress fracture of the neck of the femur is an extremely serious injury and, as the injury can have dire consequences, requires the urgent attention of an orthopaedic surgeon. Runners recovering from all stress fractures other than that of the femoral neck, should keep physically active and need to find out why the injury happened in the first place to prevent a recurrence.

As dietary calcium intake is low in runners with bone injuries, it makes sense for such runners to increase their calcium intakes but as yet there is no firm evidence that this will reduce the risk of a recurrent injury. It is generally advisable that women with menstrual disturbances should consult a specialist for advice about the need to take hormone replacement therapy if their menstrual periods do not return with a reduction in training and an increase in dietary energy intake where appropriate.

Posterior and anterior tibial and fibular bone strain ('shinsplints')

Tibial and fibular bone strain is the second most

common injury after peripatellar pain syndrome ('runner's knee'), diagnosed in distance runners. Tibial or fibular bone strain typically develops through four stages of injury. In the first stage, vague discomfort, poorly localized somewhere in the calf is noted after exercise. As training continues, the discomfort comes on during running. At first it is possible to 'run through' this pain, but if training is continued without treatment, the pain soon becomes so severe that proper training is neither enjoyable nor possible. This is a grade III injury. Ultimately, the injury may become so severe that anything more strenuous than walking is quite impossible. This grade IV bone strain injury has become a stress fracture.

In making a diagnosis of bone strain, it is important to differentiate the injury from a chronic tear in the tibialis anterior or tibialis posterior muscles. This is done by locating the site at which the greatest tenderness is felt. In bone strain injuries, this is always along either the front (anterior tibial bone strain) or back (posterior tibial bone strain) borders of the tibia or along the outside edge of the fibula (fibular bone strain). Usually the bone in the affected area has a rough corrugated feeling as a result of the build-up of a new bony (periosteal) layer at the site of the irritation. When firm finger pressure is applied to these areas, exquisite well-localized nauseating tenderness is felt.

In the early 1970s the most popular explanation for 'shinsplints' was that the tibial or fibular bone strain was caused by the build-up of pressure in one or more of the tight muscular compartments of the leg during exercise. In true tibial or fibular bone strain, however, there is no such pressure build-up and it appears that 'shinsplints' is a bone injury. Accordingly, a more accurate term for shinsplints is 'bone strain' of the named bone. The injury is caused either by excessive ankle pronation or by exposure to excessive shock to which the bone is initially unable to adapt.

The most likely explanation for most cases of tibial or fibular bone strain is that the injury occurs in bones that are undergoing remodelling in response to an increased loading stress. The response of bones to this stress has been discussed under stress fractures (a grade IV bone strain injury). Bone strain thus indicates excessive osteoclonal excavation with the development of localized or diffuse areas of bone weakness. These weaker areas are sensitive to touch, as well as to the increased loading stress of exercise.

Overstriding is thought to be the major cause of anterior tibial bone strain. Overstriding causes the forefoot to slap onto the ground and it is believed that in trying to prevent this slapping movement, the muscles in the front of the calf are forced to overwork. Ultimately, pain develops at the point where they attach to the tibia. Posterior tibial bone strain, by far the most common form of bone strain, is likely to be caused by either excessive ankle pronation or the inadequate shock-absorbing ability of bones not used to the stresses of running. It is probable that abnormal ankle pronation causes a twisting force to develop in the tibia and the fibula and that this eventually leads to minute bone cracks at the sites of greatest bone resorption, causing the pain.

Tibial and fibular bone strain is most common among five groups of athletes: middle distance high school track athletes; inexperienced joggers; competitive female runners; female aerobic dancers (especially instructors); and army recruits during their first few months of training. More experienced runners are susceptible when they start training intensively for competition. Other factors are also associated with the injury, including training errors, training surfaces and running shoes.

The typical training routine of the high school track athlete provides a perfect recipe for bone strain. Little training is done in the off-season, so that when the new season begins the athlete is exposed to an impossibly demanding training load. This usually takes the form of too much speedwork, too often, too soon, with no programming of hard/easy days (see Chapter 4). This is done under the worst possible environmental conditions of running continually in one direction on a hard unforgiving running surface, in hard uncompromising shoes. Unless the athlete has perfect lower limbs and very strong bones, the end result of bone strain or a stress fracture is predictable. Both novice and experienced distance runners who subject themselves to similar training errors of too much, too fast, too soon and wear inappropriate shoes expose themselves to similar risks.

There are also hereditary factors that predispose to most running injuries; in particular, hypermobile feet which pronate excessively and a leg-length discrepancy. In addition, there may be inadequate flexibility of the ankle caused by tight calf muscles. It is also possible that some runners may have bones that are genetically weak, which will automatically increase the risk. Other factors associated with increased risk of bone strain are muscle imbalance and flexibility, and weak bones caused by menstrual abnormalities or a low-calcium diet, or both.

Successful treatment of tibial and fibular bone strain should aim to address the cause of the injury. Once one or more of the factors outlined above have been identified as contributing to the injury; these can be addressed in an effective treatment programme. For grade I injuries which cause pain only after exercise, the first priority is to determine whether anything has changed recently in the runner's training methods. A return to previous training methods or the purchase of appropriate running shoes may be all that is required to cure the injury. If the runner pronates excessively, a strong antipronation shoe is required. If not, a softer shoe may be needed to absorb shock more effectively. Novice runners who have been running for less than 3 months can be reassured that it is likely that their injury will disappear in 4–10 weeks without any specific treatment, and even without a reduction in training. Their recovery will indicate that their bones have strengthened and adapted to the increased load. Attention must be paid to the running gait; in particular, injured runners must learn to run with a shuffle and to avoid overstriding. Another trick is to avoid pushing off with the toes, which should rather be allowed to float inside the shoe.

Another treatment option, where tight calf muscles and/or muscle imbalance have been identified, is to do specific calf muscle stretching and strengthening exercises. A specific form of treatment that can be used in all cases of bone strain is to apply ice massages to the sore areas for 20–30 min per session, 2–3 times per day. The ice should be placed in a plastic container and then massaged gently up and down the leg over the sore areas.

Women who are not menstruating regularly should, if they are knowingly restricting their food intakes, consider increasing their food intakes until normal menstrual patterns return. Alternatively, they should consult a gynaecologist for an opinion about the advisability of taking replacement oestrogen and progesterone therapy. Women who are restricting their dietary calcium intakes, usually by avoiding dairy products which provide most of the calcium in the diet, should consider taking supplementary calcium in the form of calcium tablets (500–1000 mg·day^{-1}).

When, despite trying everything listed above, pain is always present during running (grade II and III injuries), the only real hope for a cure is to acquire a corrective orthotic to wear when running. Only when the orthotic is correctly adjusted, however, will it cure the injury. If the corrective orthotic fails to provide a cure, it is likely it has not been sufficiently well designed to provide the precise degree of control required to cure the injury.

Muscle injuries

Delayed onset muscle soreness

This takes the form of that feeling of muscle discomfort that comes on 24–48 h after unaccustomed or particularly severe exercise. The diagnosis is straightforward. Muscle pain which peaks 24–48 h after exercise is indicative that the muscle has been overstressed. Persistent muscle soreness present for days and weeks on end is a strong indicator of overtraining and an absolute indicator of the need to reduce training.

The probable cause of this delayed onset muscle soreness is damage of the muscle cells, in particular the connective (supporting) tissue. Recently there have been very interesting new findings showing that there is frank disruption and death of muscle cells in athletes who complain of pronounced muscle soreness after marathon and ultra-marathon races. This damage is caused by the eccentric muscle actions of the quadriceps and calf muscles, which engage in eccentric actions each time the foot lands on the ground. Eccentric actions of these muscles are especially active particularly during downhill running. Repetitive powerful muscle contractions cause muscle cell damage by allowing calcium to accumulate inside the cells. This leads to cell death that peaks 48 h after exercise. Initiation of an inflammatory response stimulates nerve endings in the damaged tissue, causing the pain typical of delayed muscle soreness.

The only known ways to reduce muscle damage during prolonged exercise are:
• distance training;
• training downhill; and

• weight training to increase the strength of the quadriceps muscle. This type of weight training must be done with eccentric movements.

Interestingly, anti-inflammatory agents appears to have some effect in reducing delayed muscle soreness. If muscles with delayed soreness are damaged, it would seem logical that rest, with avoidance of further damaging activity, might be the best form of treatment. In fact, new studies suggest that continuing to train vigorously on muscles showing delayed soreness may delay recovery.

Chronic muscle tears

The importance of chronic (insidious) muscle tears (muscle knots) is that these are probably the third most common injury among all groups of runners and are especially common among elite runners. In addition, they are usually misdiagnosed, they can be very debilitating and they will respond only to one specific form of treatment.

There are several features in the diagnosis of muscle tears.
• The pain starts gradually, initially coming on after exercise.
• When the pain starts to occur during exercise, it is possible first to run through the pain but the pain gets progressively worse until it becomes severe enough to interfere with training. Speedwork, in particular, becomes impossible.
• The pain is almost always localized to a large muscle group, either the buttock, groin, hamstring or calf muscles.
• The pain is deep-seated and can be very severe but passes off rapidly with rest.
• It becomes difficult to push off properly with the toes if the injury is to the calf muscles.
• In contrast to bone injuries, which will improve if sufficient rest is allowed, chronic muscle tears will never improve unless the correct treatment is prescribed, so the patient can rest for months or even years without any improvement.
• To confirm that the injury is indeed a chronic muscle tear, all the runner or, preferably, a physiotherapist or other health professional need do, is to press firmly with two fingers into the affected muscle in the area in which the pain is felt. If it is possible to find a very tender hard 'knot' in the muscle, then the

injury is definitely a chronic muscle tear. It is impossible to emphasize sufficiently just how sore these knots are when palpated forcefully.

The mechanism of injury in chronic muscle tears is largely unknown but new evidence suggests that these muscle injuries occur when the muscle is contracting eccentrically. For example, the hamstring muscle is now known to tear when the muscle contracts eccentrically; that is, while it contracts but lengthens during the swing phase of the running cycle, as the muscle contracts to decelerate the foot immediately prior to heel stroke.

The calf muscle also tears during the eccentric phase of its action, immediately before the heel lifts off the ground as the knee moves forward of the ankle, so stretching the muscle eccentrically. As runners who have recurrent chronic muscle tears tend to injure the same muscles at the same site every time, usually when they start doing either more speed running or more distance training, it is probable that these tears occur at sites which are exposed to very high loading, typical of fast running.

Because the loading (exercising against an opposing force) is so concentrated over a small section of the muscle, an initial small tear develops at the site as the muscle gives way. Although the tear is initially too small to cause discomfort, once the initial tear has occurred, a cycle of repair and retear develops that leads ultimately to the large tender knot. This probably consists of muscle fibres surrounded by scar tissue.

It also seems likely that these muscles tear because they do not have sufficient eccentric strength to resist the eccentric loading imposed on them during the running stride. It follows that appropriate eccentric muscle strength should be developed in the muscles prone to chronic muscle tears in order to prevent injury.

Conventional treatment, including drugs and cortisone injections, are a waste of time in treatment of this injury. The only treatment that works is physiotherapeutic manoeuvres, including manual cross-frictions to the tender knots. If the cross-friction treatment does not induce discomfort either the diagnosis is wrong, or the physiotherapist is being too gentle.

Most chronic muscle tears respond rapidly to a few sessions of cross-frictions. The application of ultrasound treatment immediately following the cross-frictions may be of benefit. The treatment is correct if the pain while running becomes gradually less, so that progressively greater distances can be covered at a faster pace. Most injuries will require between five and 10 sessions of therapy, each lasting 5–10 min, after which most runners should be able to run entirely free of pain. Injuries that have lasted for 6 months or more may require a longer period of treatment.

As these injuries occur during eccentric muscle actions, it seems probable that strengthening the affected muscles eccentrically would reduce the risk of re-injury. Walking and running downhill backwards is a good way to load the calf muscles eccentrically. Eccentric loading of the hamstrings can best be achieved by specific exercises in the gym. These exercises must recreate the action of stopping the foot suddenly as the knee extends.

Because these injuries tend to recur, the injured runner must be fastidious about stretching the muscles that tend to be injured. This is especially important before any fast running, in particular before early morning races. Furthermore, it is essential that at the first sign of re-injury, the runner goes immediately for physiotherapy. A little treatment early on in these injuries saves a great deal of agony later.

In order to prevent chronic muscle injuries it is important that the eccentric strength of the muscles at risk of injury is increased and maintained with the appropriate eccentric strengthening programme.

Muscle cramps

Muscle cramps are defined as spasmodic painful involuntary contractions of muscles. Although muscle cramping is an important feature of some very serious muscle disorders, the cramps experienced by runners are, despite the inconvenience and discomfort they cause, usually of little medical consequence. It is clear that the propensity for cramping differs from one individual to another. Some are almost never affected, others will always develop muscle cramps if they run far enough.

Exertional cramps tend to occur in people who run further or faster than they are accustomed. Thus, the athlete whose longest regular training run is 30 km is likely to develop muscle cramps during the last few kilometres of a 42.2-km standard marathon. A novel theory holds that muscle cramps result from alterations in the sensitivity of the reflexes that originate from the muscle and tendon tension receptors. It is postulated that during prolonged exercise the inverse stretch reflex, the one that inhibits excessive muscle contraction, becomes inactive. The result is that without this protective reflex, the muscle can go into spasm (Schwellnus *et al.* 1997).

This suggests that the only factor that appears to reduce the risk of cramping is simply more training, especially long distance runs in those who run marathon and longer races. Adequate prerace stretching, attention to adequate fluid and carbohydrate replacement before and during exercise, and not running too fast too early in the race, may also be of value. Furthermore, a recent theory predicts that cramps could be prevented if the activity of the inverse stretch reflex is maintained during prolonged exercise. This is done by regularly stretching the tendons of the affected muscles. This stretching reactivates the dormant inverse stretch reflex.

The most effective form of prevention for cramps is to undertake a regular stretching programme that focuses especially on the muscles that are prone to cramp during exercise. This programme should incorporate static stretching of the affected muscles for at least 10 min a day for at least a month. Thereafter it is probable that the benefits can be maintained by a less intensive programme, perhaps 10–15 min every second day.

Tendon injuries

Achilles tendinosis

Achilles tendinosis is one of the most debilitating injuries and has curtailed the training programmes and modified the aspirations of many great and not-so-great runners. It ranks third behind anterior knee pain and bone strain in terms of frequency of occurrence in runners. It becomes increasingly common in older athletes.

Unlike muscle injuries, which are usually poorly recognized by runners and their advisers, tendon injuries do not usually present a diagnostic problem to anyone, particularly when they occur, as they usually do, in the Achilles tendon. The first indicator of injury usually comes with the first step out of bed in the morning. As soon as the afflicted foot touches the ground there is a feeling of discomfort or stiffness behind the ankle. This is usually enough to cause some initial limping which tends to wear off after a few minutes of walking. These symptoms constitute a grade I injury. If the condition is allowed to progress unchecked, discomfort may also be noted after exercise, particularly after long runs or fast intervals (grade II) and this may deteriorate gradually through grades III and IV of injury.

The most probable cause of Achilles tendinosis is that excessive ankle pronation causes a whipping action or bowstring effect in the Achilles tendon. The Achilles tendon has a relatively poor blood supply in the area in which it typically develops the injury —that is, 2–6 cm above the site of insertion of the tendon into the heel bone. It is likely that this whipping action interferes with the already tenuous blood supply to the area, leading ultimately to the death of small areas of the tendon in that region. Alternatively, a more recent explanation is that the Achilles tendon is an important shock-absorbing structure and that age and minor injury reduce its ability to absorb shock. Excessive loading, especially eccentric loading, then promotes further injury which is characterized, not by tendon inflammation (tendinitis), but by frank degeneration of the tendon cells and their supporting matrix (tendinosis). This chronic degenerative process is known as a tendinosis which further suggests that, once injured, the structure of the tendon is never again completely normal.

The injury can be brought on by any sudden increase in training distances, in particular single very long runs; too many speed sessions, particularly if these are done by running mainly on the toes; a sudden return to heavy training after lay-off; and increased inflexibility of the calf muscles caused by too much training and too little stretching.

Injuries may also be caused by shoes that:
• are heelless spikes or low-heeled shoes (racing flats);
• are worn out;
• are inappropriate to the individual runner's specific biomechanical needs;
• have a heel height of under 12–15 mm;
• have a very stiff sole and fail to bend easily at the forefoot; or
• are excessively hard and therefore increase the loading of the tendon.

Genetic factors that predispose to Achilles tendinosis include tight inflexible calf muscles, hypermobile feet and, in a small percentage of runners, the high-arched cavus or 'clunk' foot. There are possibly genetic differences in the ability of different tendons to absorb shock or to recover from the effects of heavy training and repeated eccentric loading. Age and many years of heavy training also seem to make this injury more likely. Older runners who try to train as they did in their youth appear to be at risk. This is explained by the progressive degeneration that occur in the tendon cells with increasing age.

The initial treatment for the injured Achilles tendon is to apply an ice pack to the sore area for as long as is possible each day. A suggested schedule is to apply an ice pack for at least 30 min three times per day, especially immediately before and after running. Appropriate calf muscle stretching exercises must be done for between 10 and 20 min per day. In addition, eccentric stretching of the Achilles tendon, to allow the tendon to be loaded in a stretched position, may be very helpful. This would increase the strength of the Achilles tendon during eccentric loading, such as running downhill. Although anti-inflammatory drugs and/or cortisone injections are often prescribed, they have several disadvantages.
• This treatment could suggest that a cure can be bought or swallowed. Only by learning why the injury happened will a runner ever learn how to avoid further injury.
• The money could, perhaps, be better spent on a new pair of shoes, which might have more lasting curative effects.
• There is a risk that cortisone injected into the tendon may make it more liable to rupture completely. In fact, it is very hard to condone giving a cortisone injection into the Achilles tendon. It implies buying a short-term benefit at a possible long-term cost: the risk of tendon rupture requiring emergency surgery. Furthermore, it is not clear how the anti-inflammatory effects of a cortisone injection will be of value in the treatment of a chronic degenerative condition (tendinosis). This form of treatment would be more appropriate for a chronic inflammatory condition (tendinitis) which is almost never the case in tendon injuries in runners.

When prescribing a shoe to treat Achilles tendinosis, antipronation models with rigid heel-counters and firmer mid-sole material that best reduce excessive ankle pronation should be prescribed. However, such shoes must still offer reasonable shock absorption. A 7–15-mm heel raise should be added to the running shoes, either as an addition to the heel or as firm felt material inside the running shoe. This is especially important in runners who have tight calf muscles, cavus (high-arched) feet, or leg-length inequalities.

If the Achilles tendinosis resists all treatment, then a corrective orthotic is indicated, particularly for the excessive pronator. These should be professionally made and will usually require expert readjustment before they are completely effective. It may be that an attack of Achilles tendinosis is an indication for total rest until the injury has healed. The injury can cause scarring between the Achilles tendon and its sheath which could be aggravated by continued running. But, as few runners will even consider this advice, a more acceptable approach is one of modified rest tailored to the grade of injury. One way of tailoring training to the injury is to use the 'pinch test' after each run. If the test indicates that the tendon is becoming progressively more tender after a particular training session, then this indicates either that total training should be reduced, or that that particular training session should be avoided. Alternatively, if the tendon becomes progressively less tender, then the treatment is succeeding and training distance and intensity may be gradually increased.

Physiotherapy is advised for all injuries and should be mandatory for all injuries more severe than grade I. One form of physiotherapy is cross-frictions applied to the tender areas of the tendon. This should be followed by ultrasound treatment. The ultimate danger in recurrent Achilles tendinosis is that the scarring process, which initially starts inside the tendon, progresses to involve the sheath surrounding the tendon. When this happens, adhesions (connections) are formed between the tendon and its sheath. As this happens, the free movement of the tendon inside its sheath becomes increasingly impaired and the tendon becomes susceptible to repeated attacks of tendinosis. Each of these leaves the runner progressively more debilitated until ultimately very little running is possible.

Fortunately, this injury can now be very effectively treated by a delicate surgical procedure which removes the tendon sheath together with any areas of tendon scarring. When performed by an experienced surgeon, this procedure has been shown to have a very high success rate. However, surgery should be considered only when all other techniques, including repeated sessions of cross-frictions, have been unsuccessful.

Partial or complete tear in the Achilles tendon

Two serious conditions involving the Achilles tendon need to be differentiated from Achilles tendinosis. In the partial or complete tendon ruptures, either a large portion of the tendon (partial) or the complete tendon ruptures, causing sudden dramatic pain and weakness in the affected leg. Although complete Achilles tendon rupture is an uncommon injury in distance runners, the incomplete tear frequently occurs.

The importance of recognizing complete or partial Achilles tendon ruptures is that they are conditions for which early surgery or immobilization may be indicated. Thus, if the onset of Achilles tendon pain is sudden and debilitating, unlike the gradual onset described for typical Achilles tendinosis, then it is essential that the runner seek out an experienced surgeon without delay. This must be done so that the appropriate surgery can be performed urgently. The area of torn tendon begins to degenerate shortly after injury, making surgery extremely difficult after any delay.

In a completely ruptured, and a severe partially ruptured, tendon it should be possible to feel a complete gap in the tendon. An important feature of a complete tendon rupture is that it prevents normal walking on the affected side. The runner with a completely ruptured Achilles tendon is unable to push off with that ankle, because the calf muscles that provide the power for push-off are no longer attached to the ankle by the Achilles tendon. The cause of the complete or partial tear is essentially similar to that described for Achilles tendinosis above. The partial or complete tear often occurs after a normal case of tendinosis has been aggravated, possibly by the intensification of some of the factors previously described or following a cortisone injection. If the tendon is already degenerate it is more likely to tear. Age is an important factor that makes this injury more likely. Complete immobilization on immediate surgery by a skilled orthopaedic surgeon is indicated for the partial or complete tear of the Achilles tendon.

References

Celsing, F., Blomstrand, E., Werner, B., Pihlstedt, P. & Ekblom, B. (1986) Effects of iron deficiency on endurance and muscle enzyme activity in man. *Medicine and Science in Sports and Exercise* **18**, 156–161.

Clement, D.B., Asmundson, R. & Medhurst, C.W. (1977) Haemoglobin values: comparative survey of the 1976 Canadian Olympic Team. *Canadian Medical Association Journal* **117**, 614–616.

Ledingham, I.M., MacVicar, S., Watt, I. & Weston, G.A. (1982) Early resuscitation after marathon collapse. *Lancet* **2**, 1096–1097.

Mackinnon, L.T. (1998) Future directions in exercise and immunology: regulation and integration. *International Journal of Sports Medicine* **19** (Suppl. 3), S205–S211.

Matter, M., Stittfall, T., Graves, J. *et al.* (1987) The effects of iron and folate therapy on maximal exercise performance in iron and folate deficient marathon runners. *Clinical Science* **72**, 415–422.

Maughan, R.J. (1985) Thermoregulation in marathon competition at low ambient temperature. *International Journal of Sports Medicine* **6**, 15–19.

Noakes, T.D. (1992) The hyponatraemia of exercise. *International Journal of Sports Nutrition* **2**, 205–228.

Noakes, T.D. (1993) Fluid replacement during exercise. *Exercise and Sports Science Reviews* **21**, 297–330.

Peters, J. (1955) *In the Long Run*. Cassell, London.

Scheffer, A.L. & Austen, K.F. (1980) Exercise-induced anaphylaxis. *Journal of Allergy and Clinical Immunology* **66**, 106–111.

Schwellnus, M.P., Derman, E.W. & Noakes, T.D. (1997) Aetiology of skeletal muscle 'cramps' during exercise: a novel hypothesis. *Journal of Sports Sciences* **15**, 277–285.

Siegel, A.J. (1980) Exercise-induced anaphylaxis. *Physician and Sports Medicine* **8**, 95–98.

Recommended reading

Noakes, T.D. (1991) *Lore of Running*, 3rd edn. Human Kinetics, Champaign, Illinois.

Noakes, T.D. & Granger, S. (1996) *Running Injuries*, 2nd edn. Oxford University Press, Cape Town.

Index

7/01

DATE DUE

#47-0108 Peel Off Pressure Sensitive